MIRACULOUSLY MY OWN

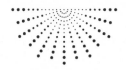

SAMANTHA J MORGAN

PURPOSEFUL INK PRESS

Published by Purposeful Ink Press, PO Box 877 Rogersville, MO 65742

Scripture taken from the HOLY BIBLE, NEW INTERNATIONAL VERSION. Copyright C 1973, 1978, 1984 International Bible Society. Used by permission of Zondervan Bible Publishers.

When noted scripture taken from THE MESSAGE Copyright 1993, 1994,1995, 2000, 2001, 2002. Used by permission of NavPress Publishing Group.

Details in some pieces of the story have been changed to protect the identities of the persons involved.

Front cover photo by Jamie Moore Photography

Cover by Amanda Walker PA and Design

Insert photos courtesy of Samantha J Morgan

Back cover author photo by Lindsey Leggett, All Sides Photography

ISBN: 978-1-7358545-0-2 (Paperback)

978-1-7358545-1-9 (e-book)

978-1-7358545-2-6 (Hardcover)

To my son,
We traveled the world to find you, but God handpicked the best
boy in the whole world just for me. I love your tender heart and
your big brown eyes that seek to please me and your dad.
Always know, just like the love of Christ, you never have to earn
my love. I am proud of you, I love you, and I will always say,
"That's my boy!"

Love you always Rush boy,
Mom

Not flesh of my flesh
    Nor bone of my bone,
    But still miraculously my own.
    Never forget for a single minute,
    You didn't grow under my heart
    But in it.

— FLEUR CONKLING HEYLIGER

INTRODUCTION

My journey from infertility to adoption was difficult and littered with pain and uncertainty. It was also filled with the promises of God. In the most difficult times of our journey, I clung to Romans 8:26-28 from the Message Bible.

"Meanwhile, the moment we get tired in the waiting, God's Spirit is right alongside helping us along. If we don't know how or what to pray, it doesn't matter. He does our praying in and for us, making prayer out of our wordless sighs, our aching groans. He knows us far better than we know ourselves, knows our pregnant condition, and keeps us present before God. That's why we can be so sure that every detail in our lives of love for God is worked into something good."

I wrote on a scrap piece of paper that I still keep tucked in my Bible today; "Keep my eyes on God, not the end results I want, and I will be AMAZED by the outcome." I was and still am today amazed by our outcome! I hope our story encourages you to trust God's plan for your own Journey. Even when you can't see the ending.

Love and support,
Samantha

CHAPTER ONE

"NO, absolutely not, I don't want someone else's problem!" Michael said, "My mom has worked in social services for years. I've heard all the stories."

"I understand, Michael. I hear you, but I want to know all of our options." I was getting nowhere.

"I want a family too, someday. If that's what you want, but we're going to be okay. With or without kids. I didn't marry you to reproduce." I exhaled, knowing he loved me more than anything; even more than the one thing I should be able to give him. At that moment, I realized I was being harder on myself than anyone.

"I'm tired of people asking us when we're having kids. Like it's some kind of joke. Like we don't want them," I said.

"It's no one's business when we have kids, Samantha."

I lowered my head, "Why is this happening, why us? What did we do to deserve this? It's not fair every twenty-year-old can get pregnant. I'm twenty-eight, you're thirty-three; we aren't getting any younger."

Michael moved closer, lifting my chin, "Life's not fair Samantha, and if we didn't live in small-town Missouri where the average age of getting pregnant was twenty-two, then you wouldn't feel so bad. We aren't that old, and there are far worse things that could be happening to us than this. Someone is getting a cancer diagnosis with six months to live right now. It's not the end of the world if we can't have kids." He looked straight into my eyes, "We have to stop asking, 'Why us?' and start asking, 'Why not us?' We can handle this." His arms held me tight, "We can handle this. Let's give it a few months. You're stressed and thinking desperately. You may want to look into in vitro later; we don't have to decide this second."

"I want to look into adoption too. Okay? Will you at least consider it?" I asked as tears filled my eyes. He nodded, but I wasn't convinced he meant it. At least the seed was planted.

The doctor's heartless words were still on my mind, "I'm sorry, but the sun and the moon and the stars would have to align for you and your husband to get pregnant. In vitro fertilization is your best option." I was tired. Tired of treatments, tired of fertility doctors, and I was tired of the ups and downs of this infertility rollercoaster.

My best friend in infertility, Jamie, and her husband Nate had been actively trying IVF. It had not been fun to watch. She shared the pain of the procedures, the scheduling nightmare, and the toll it took on her emotionally. All of that and they still had no baby.

I heard a coworker at school tell Jamie, after a failed IVF cycle, "Well, now you just get to have fun practicing at home!" This made my blood boil. There was nothing fun about scheduled sex, internal ultra sounds, and self-administered injections. No one understands infertility unless they have experienced it, and that's part of the reason I kept it to myself. If it weren't for Jamie, I would have completely lost it by now. Having at least one person to talk to that truly understood was priceless.

Did God intend for us to try every possible avenue to create a child? The more I thought about in vitro, the more turned off I became. It could cost upwards of 20,000 dollars. That's money we didn't have, and I didn't even know if I could get pregnant. My mental state was rocky; I needed some kind of guarantee, not a shot in the dark. The chances of us doing IVF with no success and spending all that money were high. Money that we could use toward adoption. *That could be God's plan too, right?* Jamie and Nate were going to explore foster care. Maybe adoption could be a good thing.

Michael was definitely not on board, and even though I was scared, I felt pulled in that direction. He just needed more time; and I needed to talk with Joy.

"Elkanah her husband would say to her, 'Hannah, why are you weeping? Why don't you eat? Why are you downhearted? Don't I mean more to you than ten sons?'"
1 Samuel 1:8

THE LIFE of a pastor's wife is never her own. I felt bad for bothering her, but I didn't trust anyone else with this information. My mother, of course, would normally be my go-to, but I knew she would worry and fret herself sick. No, Joy was the perfect friend to share this sensitive information with. She would have realistic, Godly advice.

I pulled into the church parking lot to find Joy already waiting. When we talked on the phone, I only explained that I had some life issues I needed help with, and Joy was more than willing to drop what she was doing to meet me. She gave more of herself than she took, and I appreciated and valued her advice. She was always realistic and to the point, and that is exactly what I needed.

"Hello, friend!" Joy smiled as she walked toward the church.

"Hi," I gave a tired smile back.

"So, how are you?"

I smiled, "Oh, you know the usual life crisis. Sorry to bother you!"

Joy tilted her head to look at me from over her glasses, "How are you, really?" Joy always knew just how to get to the point.

"Well, I haven't shared this with many, so if this could stay between us?"

"Absolutely," Joy said.

"Michael and I have been trying to have a baby for years now," pinching my lips together, I gathered my thoughts. Admitting it out loud was harder than I expected. Air filled my lungs as Joy patiently waited, "We pretty much got an ultimatum from the doctor to forget about kids or do in vitro." Pinching the bridge of my nose didn't help; the tears fell. "Joy, I don't know where God is. I don't know why he has forgotten me."

"Oh, Samantha," Joy's hug felt like a warm towel from the dryer. "I am so sorry! But that doesn't mean God has left you!"

I was relieved to hear her reaction, "I know how it hurts when you want something so bad but it never comes, or you can't see the 'why' in God's timing. I have to say, I kind of know how you feel. We were never able to have more kids after Kaitlyn. We tried and tried, prayed and prayed, and it just never happened."

"I didn't know!" I was so thankful to be understood. "In vitro scares me to death. I just always believed God would make it happen for us, you know?" As the past four years poured out of my heart, I started to breathe easier, to see more clearly. I released the pressure cooker of emotions that had been building for years. By the end, we were both sobbing.

"So I just don't know what to do next," I said.

"You don't have to know what to do right now, you

know that you love God, you can control that, but you cannot control or predict Him. Why would we even bother to worship a God we have all figured out? What kind of God would He be?" Joy smiled. "You will make a great mom one day, God will make a way."

"For in this hope we were saved. But hope that is seen is no hope at all. Who hopes for what they already have? But if we hope for what we do not yet have, we wait for it patiently."
Romans 8:24-25

JOY WAS SPOT ON. Why would I want to worship a God I could predict? Michael was right too, this wasn't the worst that could happen to us. But in vitro? Is that what God intended, for us to create a child at all costs? Then, to not even know if it would work in the end.

I grappled with my thoughts the whole way home, weighing the options and praying for God to speak. So clearly, as if God himself asked me the question, I said out loud, "Do I want to be pregnant or do I want to be a mom?"

Pregnancy lasts nine months, but being a mom lasts a lifetime. Deep down, I had always known the answer. I just wanted to be a mom. To nurture and shape a child's life, to feel needed and give unconditional love, to protect and raise a child's soul. I just wanted to be a mom. But Michael, he wasn't there yet. So I prayed.

Jesus, I need you now more than ever. I can't do this alone. I am ready to surrender to your plan, not my own. Please God, take the desire of pregnancy away. If it's never meant to be, please take it away. Take away the bitterness and place in me a new heart, a new longing for something more. Soften Michael's heart to the idea of adoption. Open doors for him. Show him your love in adoption. And, please Lord, guide me, help me research and confirm this is your plan for us.

I dove headfirst into researching adoption. The more I searched, the more my heart ached for these children. So much like me, needing and praying for a family, yet they were far more vulnerable and helpless to their own situation. Foster care, domestic, international. There were so many options for adoption and so many orphaned children in the world. I had no idea.

"Look at this, Michael." I turned the computer to face him. "Did you know there are nearly 443,000 children in foster care? Thirteen thousand just in Missouri!"

He looked a bit taken aback, "Really?"

"Yes, there are photo listings of children available right now. What if we tried fostering first, just to see?"

"I don't know, Samantha. Are you sure you could keep a child and then give them back? Have you thought more about in vitro?"

"I'm not doing in vitro." The finality in my voice surprised even me.

"Alright. That's fine, but I'm still trying to picture what

adoption would be like. I'm just having a hard time wrapping my head around it."

"Okay, but be honest. Have you ever really thought about how many kids didn't have parents?"

"No, I guess not."

"Adoption is bigger than ourselves. Like you said, 'There are worse things than not having children.' Like not having parents!"

Michael smirked, knowing I had stopped that argument with his own words. I prayed in my heart for God to keep working.

Jesus, I am ready. I'm ready to go where you take us. Please God, soften Michael's heart. Show him what adoption can feel and look like. And please guide me, show me where our baby is.

CHAPTER TWO

M ichael and I were both teachers. We were mandated reporters. We were around kids all day long, but I never knew the true problems they faced. Sure, there were the kids who didn't have as much as others, didn't have help with their homework, or were disruptive in class. It wasn't until I truly started researching that I found the staggering statistics that were our foster care system.

In the state of Missouri, there were 19,400 children in foster care. This broke my heart; not just for Missouri, but for kids in every state and every country in the world. If it was that bad in Missouri, I couldn't imagine what it was like in other countries. These children needed homes. They needed parents and stability; foster care seemed like the next logical step to adoption.

"And whoever welcomes a little
child like this in my name welcomes me."
Matthew 18:5

FRANTIC WOULD HAVE BEEN AN UNDERSTATEMENT. Everything had to be perfect. I even cleaned the oven and refrigerator. I still couldn't believe Michael agreed to this meeting. He said he was just doing this for me, but I knew God was working on him. He had been listening and asking questions as I watched adoption videos on YouTube. I could tell he was coming around, but God still needed to work a miracle in his heart.

"My goodness, would you slow down?" Michael said from the couch.

"Would you go change your shirt?" I yelled from the bathroom as I finished my makeup.

"What's wrong with my shirt?" he huffed. I didn't answer, he knew it was just an old t-shirt. "Oh, alright. I'll change it, but don't expect me to change my pants too!"

I laughed to myself, "He thinks he's so tough."

"I heard that!" he yelled back.

Our apartment was so small, barely 600 square feet, but we had land and were building our dream home. The house we would raise our children in. It would have a basement and five bedrooms; one of the rooms attached to the master bedroom would be the nursery. Of course, this dream was before the diagnosis of infertility, but we were building it in faith that one day it would be full of kids.

I checked off my mental to-do list. *Vacuum, check. Bed made, check. Yard mowed, check. Toilets, windows, mirrors. Check. Check. Check. Would she look in the storage closet outside?*

I had called Social Services to inquire about foster parenting. They were more than happy to set up an appointment at our home to see if our living conditions were suitable. I didn't exactly know what that meant, but I assumed whoever came would want a tour of our home. I wanted to know all I could about every option to adopt, and foster care was the first on my list.

A knock on the door snapped me back to reality. I was frazzled from cleaning and getting ready, making everything look perfect, including Michael and myself. This was a big step for him, so I needed this to go better than perfect.

"Are you going to open the door?" Michael stood looking at me. Exhaling, I turned the handle.

"Hi, come on in!" I plastered a smile and greeted her.

"Hello, I'm Jodi." She shook my hand.

"I'm Samantha, and this is Michael." Michael nodded and extended his hand. We sat on the loveseat, and Jodi took the chair. Our little apartment was too small for a full couch. It had one bedroom, a second room I'd call the master closet, and one tiny bathroom. I mean, the washing machine was in the kitchen and the dryer was in the outside carport closet. It was that small. I was so worried about what she would think, but I explained that our new home would have plenty of room and would be finished within the year.

Jodi got right to work as she opened her folder of paperwork and began the to-do list. She tackled the work like we had already accepted the mission. The stack of paperwork was passed off to me as I sat staring.

"I know it looks like a lot, but that doesn't all have to be done right now. The application is on top. You need to sign off on a background check and get fingerprinted soon before you can move forward. Oh, and there is a medical evaluation that will need to be filled out by your doctor." She spoke quickly as I took mental notes.

"So, this would need to be finished before starting classes?" I asked.

"Yes, most definitely," she answered, still shuffling through her papers. "You have to pass all the evaluations and background checks before thirty hours of class."

"So once we finish classes, how soon can we adopt?" I got right to the point.

"Adopt? Well, that may or may not happen. Our main goal is always to reunify children with biological parents or family."

"So there isn't a process for those that want to only adopt through foster care?" I asked.

"These kids need a place to stay, hopefully short term, anywhere from a few weeks to a few years sometimes. If parents don't cooperate and there is no other family, the case could end with adoption. It could happen, and it does happen, but those cases can get dragged out for months, sometimes years. I can't lead you to believe this would be the best avenue to adoption." She went on, "There are always older children who are available for adoption, but you two are pretty young to jump into raising a teenager."

"I see, well, do you need to look at the house?" I could tell she was looking around, sizing up our home.

"Yes, I'll just take a quick look around for my notes." It wasn't large enough for us both, so I kept my seat next to Michael as I motioned her on toward the small hallway.

"Through there is our bedroom, and the second bedroom I use as a closet. The bathroom is at the end."

Jodi stood in the hall surveying the remainder of our tiny house. "Oh, I see your water heater is open to the hall, that won't work. Do you have a carbon monoxide detector?"

"No, we don't." I said as Michael elbowed me in the ribs. I didn't even turn to acknowledge him.

"That is something you will have to have," she said, writing on her notepad as she walked back a few steps to the living room. "Your house is small, but we could get you started with classes. You could have one child at a time until you move. The only problem is they come in sibling groups a lot of the time."

Michael looked on from the loveseat, obviously done with it all. I knew exactly what he was thinking. "Okay, well, thank you for coming. We have a lot to talk about." I was ready to end this meeting. As I stood to open the door for Jodi, my heart sank to the floor. God himself was closing this door. Adopting through foster care could take years if it ever happened at all, and Jodi hadn't given me much hope that this journey would end with adoption. Maybe someday we would be ready to foster, but adoption was my main goal; my heart was so very fragile.

Lord, I just want to be a mom. Have a child share our last name. A child that calls me Mama. If not this, then what's next Jesus?

"Think about it and be in touch when you're ready to start classes!" Jodi waved as she headed out the door. I turned slowly, resting my head on the door to close it the rest of the way. I already knew what was coming.

"Are you kidding me?" Michael started, "The regulations for this are out of control. Fire extinguishers, carbon monoxide detectors, no strings on the window shades. It seems to me..."

"I know, I know, I agree with you," I assured him.

"You do?" He looked suspicious.

"I do. This isn't for us. I knew what you were thinking the whole time. I want kids that need forever parents. These poor kids are trapped in limbo between their parents getting their act together and the government wanting control of them. We wouldn't even qualify at this point with our house being so small. She gave us a list a mile long of things we would have to get or change. The more she talked, the more I felt this was not for us."

"Well, good. I was afraid you were sold on this idea, and I wasn't ready to show the woman my underwear drawer!" we chuckled at his little joke. This felt like a step backwards for Michael, but at least we could still laugh together.

"He will yet fill your mouth with laughter
and your lips with shouts of joy."
Job 8:21

CHAPTER THREE

"I just met the most amazing girl!" Michael said.

"Hold up, you met another girl? I thought I was the only girl for you?" I grinned. He kissed my cheek and smiled.

"A different girl. Did you know Tim and Lora adopted a little girl?"

"What? Who? Where have you been?" I asked, still confused by his excitement.

Michael poured out his day about meeting with our insurance agent, Tim. Tim was a guy's guy, and Michael had always admired him. He liked talking about cars, sports, and business.

"Lora was out of the office today, so when I went back to Tim's office there was this little girl playing on the floor. Finally, curiosity got the best of me." Michael was talking fast, "I thought he only had older boys, but that's when he told me they had adopted."

I stood in awe of my husband. He was truly taken with this little girl. All the research I was doing must have been pulling on his heart, but this meeting showed him what I had been praying for. That he might see what adoption could look like, but was he ready to commit?

"I told Tim about us not getting pregnant and stuff. I hope that was ok?" Michael asked.

"Yes, of course," I was too happy to care.

"I don't know all the details, but I know Lora flew over there to meet her and pick her up."

"Ok, slow down. So you are okay with adopting now?" I asked.

"Samantha, I wanted kids to make you happy, but after meeting Lisette, her name is Lisette by the way, I just realized kids are just little people. It's not fair we couldn't have kids, but it's even more unfair to be a child without a home." Michael said, "and to be honest I've been more scared about being a dad than anything." And with that, my prayers had been answered in so many ways.

"I'm sorry we can't have kids, but I don't want to deny you children through adoption either." My heart swelled at his words as I thanked God for this miracle. My sweet Jesus had used the most normal of days to change Michael's mind and heart. All the talking in the world would not have convinced him. It took the right person at the right time, and God knew just who and when that would be.

"Carry each other's burdens, and in this way
you will fulfill the law of Christ."
Galatians 6:2

INFERTILITY HAD CHANGED ME. I was the same person as before, just sad. Everything had been clouded with sadness. Holidays and family gatherings, Mother's Day at church was the worst. I didn't want to be like this. I didn't want infertility to define me, but deciding together that adoption was God's plan made life feel lighter. My outlook changed, I could see a future. Not one I had imagined, but one God had planned for us. As we talked about what would come next, I knew we needed to narrow down what type of adoption to do and find an agency.

Barrenness would not hold me back from becoming a mother. Giving my infertility to God allowed me to get out of His way. He can take the bad that life throws at us, and He always has a solution. This had always been His plan.

"We have a few things to figure out, Michael." I started the conversation again.

Adoption consumed life itself. I woke up thinking about it, I daydreamed about my kids, I researched agencies every day, watched videos about adoption, read parenting books about it, and fell asleep at night dreaming about it. I knew Michael wasn't consumed with it, but I

was so thankful he was on board and actively partic-
ipating.

"Okay, what do we need to figure out?" he asked.

"If we have ruled out foster care for now…" I started.

"For now?" Michael stopped me.

"Yes, for now. That leaves domestic adoption and international," I finished. Michael nodded for me to continue. "They both have pros and cons, in my opinion. The biggest difference is how we get picked for the children and their age. Whether we use an agency or not, domestically we wait for a birth mom to choose us."

"So… a baby?" Michael looked worried.

"Yes, a baby. We could be at the delivery and be involved as much as the birth mom wanted."

"And you would want a baby?" Michael asked.

"It would be nice, yes, but not necessarily. I think I'm open to a little older, but like we talked about with the social worker, I don't think I'm ready to raise a teenager. I don't want to be selfish, but I do want to experience what every other new mom does. As young as possible would be nice."

"What do you think about international?" he asked. "It's so sad knowing there are kids in orphanages across the world, and they have little chance of getting out."

"The cost is more," I said.

"I just keep thinking about Lisette and my conversation with Tim about the condition of these orphanages." Michael was still so impressed with Lisette.

"I'm good with looking deeper into international

adoption. That helps with not being at the mercy of someone choosing us. We would be getting referrals of children instead. I would have a little more control, I guess. So, how many kids do we want?" I smiled.

"What do you mean how many? One, right? People start with one at a time!" Michael thought I was kidding.

"Most of the time, but if we adopt internationally, it would be nice to have siblings. That way they have a connection. I don't want to take a child out of all they have ever known and expect them to love us for it."

"You have thought more about this than you let on. We aren't talking about babies right?" Michael asked.

"No, no babies. Maybe toddlers, even up to five years old," I had done my research.

"I'm leaning toward international then, because honestly, I wouldn't know what to do with a baby," Michael admitted.

"I would just want them to have something familiar to help them adjust, and adopting siblings would be the best. Right?"

"I would be okay with that. We get two and done?" Michael said.

"Maybe," I winked. "I might want more." Michael just smirked at me. "These applications also make you select health issues we would accept or not."

"That's up to our health insurance. We can't bring a child home if we can't afford his medical needs." Michael said that as non-negotiable, but I knew he was right.

"What country are you leaning toward?" I asked.

"I thought everyone adopted from Africa or China until I met Lisette." Michael hadn't thought too much into this. "You know, Tim said we could go out to dinner one night. You can talk to his wife Lora about it and meet Lisette."

"I think that's a great idea!

"I will not leave you as orphans; I will come to you. Before long, the world will not see me anymore, but you will see me. Because I live, you also will live."
John 14:18-19

AFRICA, Asia, South America, Central America; the world was the limit. I looked at all the options, from wait time to children available. It helped to narrow down countries that were a part of the Hague Convention, a treaty to prevent child abduction from one country to another.

After months of narrowing down countries, eastern Europe was still on our radar. I researched agencies, and Russia stayed at the top of the list. Michael's meeting with Lisette kept coming up, and the number of people adopting from Russia were less than other popular countries. Most of all, we couldn't shake the thought of these kids aging out and being marked as an orphan the rest of their life.

We learned that everyone in Russia has an ID card, much like a driver's license here in the states. But there, when a child ages out of an orphanage, they don't get a fresh start or a chance to change their circumstances. No, in Russia, their ID card is marked ORPHAN for the rest of their life, determining what jobs they can have. College is definitely out. The majority of them end up in prostitution or dealing drugs instead of sweeping streets.

My search narrowed to finding an agency that worked in Russia and had a good reputation. I requested information packets from every agency, and the huge envelopes started rolling in. I combed through every one, comparing the cost and looking up each of them on the Better Business Bureau. As my pile of potential agencies got smaller, I started making phone calls to talk with case workers. I wanted an agency that would be compassionate and caring that this was our first adoption. I wanted someone that would walk me through the process and answer all my questions and fears. After talking with several agencies, I found Adoption Associates Inc. I didn't feel like just a number, and they had been established in Russia for years.

We agreed siblings from Russia were doable for us. We knew the living conditions there and the future they faced. They would need us as much as we needed them. With our agency application filled out and the first fee paid, we were ready for a wild ride. The home study lay ahead, and I understood why people call adoption 'birth by paperwork'. We had just begun with background checks and interviews, and the agency said it could take three to six months to finish. Medical evaluations, phycological evaluations, financial evaluations, and home inspections would come. Once the home study was finished, it needed to be translated into Russian. All of that, with our visas and travel documents, would be combined into what they called a dossier and sent to Russia. It was all a little overwhelming.

"When you pass through the waters, I will be with you; and when you pass through the rivers, they will not sweep over you. When you walk through the fire , you will not be burned; the flames will not set you ablaze."
Isaiah 43:2

CHAPTER FOUR

I pulled up to Mom and Dad's and let myself in, as always, without knocking.

"Mom, are you home?" I yelled up the stairs.

"I'll be right down, hon," Mom yelled back. The time had come to tell our families. I wondered how she would respond. My children would be the first grandkids, unless my older brother surprised us. Curtis was married, and my little brother Clayton was getting close. As the first to marry, I'm sure everyone was wondering what was taking us so long. My parents always laughed saying they were too young to be called grandma and grandpa. They never wanted to pressure us to have kids, but I wondered if they were ready.

"Hey!" Mom said as she came down the stairs.

"So I have some news for you," I started.

"Okay, do you need anything to drink?" Mom smiled and headed for the dining room table.

"No, I'm good." The dining table had withstood three kids, birthday parties and family gatherings, a house remodel, and long division lessons. She was going to be shocked, maybe upset, that I had kept this from her for too long, but I had good reasons. Mom was always cautious. We weren't allowed to have a trampoline as kids, because she was sure we would break an arm. I was keeping her heart from worry.

"This may be a little surprising, but Michael and I have decided to adopt. We haven't had any luck getting pregnant." I got it out in one timid breath.

Just as quickly, Mom said, "What? How long have you been trying?" her eyes were as big as saucers, even though I warned her.

"Several years."

"Well, I've never heard this. Have you tried everything?"

"I'm not asking for permission. I'm telling you we're adopting, we've been trying for over four years. We just never shared all the details with you. I didn't want you to worry." I knew it would take Mom time to process this kind of news, much like myself.

"Oh, honey, I'm so sorry. I had no idea, I just want to fix it for you," she said.

"It's okay. I don't need fixed. Really. I just need you on my side. This has been heartbreaking for us, but I'm finally excited again. There was no sense in both of us stressed and worried. We've already started the process to adopt two kids from Russia."

"TWO? RUSSIA?" Mom sounded shocked again, "Why Russia?"

"That's where my kids are, and that's where God has your grandbabies."

"For God did not give us a spirit of timidity, but a spirit of power, of love and of self-discipline."
2 Timothy 1:7

AS THE DAYS and weeks progressed, the whole family became so excited. I knew Mom's initial reaction would be to protect me, but now that it was happening, they were excited.

"What do you want to be called?" I asked with a laugh. "Glamma, MiMi, Mam-ma, GIGI? We could call Dad Poppi!"

"Nope, Grandma and Grandpa are just fine." Mom smiled with a wink.

This would be the last Christmas for just me and Michael. After this year, I wouldn't let another go by without kids. It was going to happen. God was going to make it happen. The home study would be finished soon, and then the dossier paperwork that is sent overseas could get started. Each step allowed me to mark things off the to-do list. This Christmas was also the time to share the news with the rest of the family. Michael's parents were so excited for us. Michael's older brother had children, so ours would just add more grandchildren. Christmas dinner would be a perfect time to share with the extended family.

"So we have some news we would like to share with everyone," I started. My mother-in-law beamed with excitement. The aunts, uncles, and cousins all looked our way with the knowing faces of a pregnancy announcement. All the cousins were grown, married, and toting children of their own.

I looked at Michael and smiled. His smile and nod encouraged me. "Michael and I are adopting!" I scanned the room for reactions.

"WHAT, that is awesome!" Uncle Gary was up and hugging my neck and shaking Michael's hand.

"We thought you were going to say you were pregnant!" Aunt Debbie laughed, "So tell us more!"

I went on to share about struggling with infertility and the journey to adoption. I shared our excitement of possibly having two kids home by next Christmas. They had so many questions, and I oddly enjoyed opening up about the whole process.

"The dossier packet is next. That just means our home study is getting translated and ready to send to Russia. We have some government paperwork to fill out too, federal background checks, but after that we go on the waiting list!"

"This is just great guys! I'm so happy for you!"

"We can't wait to meet them!"

"What exciting news!" The whole family was so happy for us! After hearing everyone's reactions, I didn't know why we kept things a secret for so long, but deep down, I knew it was fear. The fear of rejection. The devil loves to use that against me.

With both of our families excited and prepared, we had finished our home study just in time to relax for Christmas, and finally, we had an appointment for federal fingerprinting and background clearance. A quick trip to St. Louis to finish it up, and then our visas would be approved.

"Was that not the craziest thing you have ever done?" I brought up the psychological evaluation again.

"It was a little creepy. I'd never been in a shrink's office before. I'm glad he didn't figure out you were crazy." Michael never took his eyes off the road, waiting for my reaction.

"Hmm, yeah. I just knew they would think I was crazy for marrying you, ya jerk!" I punched his shoulder. "It took way longer than I thought. I expected maybe an hour, and to split us up separately before we talked to him together."

"I'm glad the medicals are done. We don't have to do any of that while we are there, right? I'd hate to give blood in a Russian hospital," Michael said.

"We shouldn't. I'm so tired of all the hoops and paper-work. Needing a doctor to sign this, an accountant to sign that, the government to approve it all." Having the dossier finished and paperwork all done would make a great Valentines Day present.

The dossier was wrapping up and didn't take as long to translate as I thought it would. It was so thick, looking more like a college thesis paper. No more fingerprinting, medical tests, psych evaluations. Now we waited for a referral.

CHAPTER FIVE

We weren't completely finished with our dossier or funding when the first referral came in. It came much sooner than expected.

"Hello, Morgans," our agency worker, Oksana, said. Having our phone on speaker was getting normal as we both replied, "Hello."

"I have referral for you. I know you wanted two children, but a boy just came to us, and we wanted to give you option," Oksana explained.

"Okay, how does this work? Do we get an email?" I asked.

"Yes, I have just emailed to you," Oksana said.

With a thank you and a goodbye, I couldn't wait to check. We took a deep breath and pressed open. The greeting letter was much of the same, but attached was the referral. We opened the document to one page of information about a little boy. His developmental and medical information was sparse, but it was his picture that concerned us both. It was an old picture and very grainy. We felt something was off.

There were plenty of mixed feelings. I felt bad to say no, but this didn't feel right. We didn't have all of our funds in order yet, and our paperwork wasn't complete either. We felt rushed, and had a small inkling that this boy might not be real, or possibly older. I was also worried what turning this referral down would do to our wait time, but ultimately, we decided he wasn't for us.

---

*"For the Holy Spirit will teach you at
that time what you should say."*
Luke 12:12

OUR DOSSIER HAD BEEN SENT off and months had gone by with no referral. School was coming to an end, and I had my mind set on a restful summer. This year had been crazy, and I was ready for a change, even if it was only a change in seasons. Most everyone knew we were adopting; there was satisfaction in the truth. That saying, 'the truth shall set you free' was so true.

Even though we were waiting, it was a peaceful wait. I was truly happy again. We knew our time would come, my only concern would be updating the home study and dossier if we had to wait over a year.

Lord, if you could make this happen before our one year mark, that would be great! I said a quick prayer. While my students were away at P.E., I checked my phone and was surprised to see a voicemail. I pressed the button and waited.

"Hello, Samantha, we are sending you email containing a referral for brother/sister sibling group. Take a look and tell me if you have any questions." I laid the phone down, saving the voice message from Oksana; with a few clicks, I was staring at the email.

A tug of war broke out in my mind. Should I open it now or wait to open it with Michael? I was so excited, it was hard to wait, but I knew I should. Well, maybe just a peek wouldn't hurt.

When the school bell rang, my bag was already packed. As soon as the school buses pulled out, so did I, and I made it home in record time.

I barely stopped as I swung open the door, "Michael, where are you? We have a referral! Michael?"

"I'm right here, slow down," he laughed.

"I've been waiting all day to open this!"

"And I'm supposed to believe you didn't look?" he laughed again, knowing me all too well.

"Okay, I looked at their pictures. That's it," holding up my right hand with a grin. "I promise. They are so cute, Michael."

"Well, let's open it. We need to look at the medical

information and everything before you get too attached," he said.

I knew all of that, but still my heart knew it didn't matter what the medicals said. I had already fallen in love with those faces. The dream of becoming a mother was so close. We opened the email, together this time, skipping the long medical information until their pictures filled the screen. I paused, letting Michael process what was about to happen.

"Look at those little faces, Michael!" I finally said.

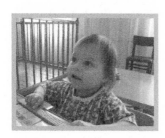

"Okay, they're cute, and he looks like a little tank," Michael agreed.

"He looks sad to me," I said with such a yearning to comfort him.

"Let's look at the medicals and information before you get attached," Michael said logically.

Yegor and Krishina were full siblings, just as we had asked for. Yegor, the oldest, was three and a half, and his little sister would be two in the fall. There were no glaring red flags, but their pictures were sad.

Yegor's rounded face showed years of living in a very different world. *Were they mistreated?* The corners of his lips drifted down like his eyes. Beautiful brown eyes against

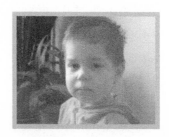

his pale skin. *Did he get the attention he needed? Enough food to eat each day?* His brown hair had just been wet and combed over, but was thinner than a three-year-old's hair should be, possibly signs of malnourishment.

Krishina was tiny, but had a brighter look upon her face. Her green eyes and olive skin had more color than Yegor's, and her hair was just about as thick as his. Swallowed whole by her clothes, she was so tiny. But at only a year and a half, there was still hope in her eyes.

These kids were not plan B. Once I allowed God to write my motherhood story, they became plan A. Our first choice. We could have tried in vitro and done more to have biological children, and that would have been fine if that's where God wanted us. But it wouldn't have felt right.

Lord, cover my babies with your protection. Keep them safe until I can reach them. I pray for their caregivers, and all the children needing a home, but let my babies be their favorite.

"So are you ready?" I asked Michael.

"Yes, let's do it." Michael kissed my forehead. It was still business hours, so I didn't wait to call our agency.

"We are ready to move forward with Yegor and Krishina," I spoke to Oksana.

"Wonderful news, just wonderful," she said. "I will email you travel agent. That is something you need not to worry about as you go."

"Thank you so much. We are so excited!" I hung up the phone and smiled. This was happening, really happening.

"So when do we leave? What's next?" Michael asked.

"Oh, crap, I don't know. I was too excited to ask anything," I chuckled. "I'm sure Oksana will send us an email."

"Though the mountains be shaken and the hills be removed, yet my unfailing love for you will not be shaken nor my covenant of peace be removed, says the Lord, who has compassion on you."
Isaiah 54:10

COMMUNICATION with the agency happened weekly, sometimes daily. We wouldn't be leaving until the end of August or beginning of September. Not the best time for teachers to be gone, but we didn't get to choose.

The travel agent was arranging airfare. It would take us four different flights to get to Kaliningrad, Russia, losing time as we traveled across eight different time zones.

Summer flew by with preparation, and the new school year was upon us. Planning for a new year was always stressful, but the added stress of preparing for weeks of a substitute was awful. It had to be done, and I was excited for the reason to be doing it. We were just weeks away from meeting our kids, and I wanted to be able to stay in touch with family and friends, so I made a private Facebook group.

AUGUST 25

Michael and I would like to share our adoption journey with family and close friends. This was the best way to keep in contact with people on our trip. We will be leaving for Russia September 3rd to meet Yegor and Krishina. Your prayers will be greatly appreciated!!!

CHAPTER SIX

Camcorder in hand to record every moment, a laptop stowed away to communicate with family, and I had the feeling that God was finally on our side.

Dear Heavenly Father, thank you for this opportunity and these children. Watch over us as we travel and cover us with your protection. Keep my babies healthy and well taken care of. Bless the caretakers watching them and make my kids their favorite.

September 2

We're off. I'll post something as soon as we can! Leave St. Louis 11:20 in the morning! We should get there at 1:00p.m. Missouri time Sunday.

WE WERE HEADING TO RUSSIA, and I was walking on clouds. This was our first international flight, and the first time leaving the safety of the United States. It was an adventure of a lifetime, and to think, I would be meeting my future children in just a few days. Family and friends were so excited for us. Out of boredom from a five hour layover in Helsinki, Finland, I took advantage of the airport Wi-Fi to keep our family and friends updated. I had no idea how often I would be able to post to the Facebook group.

September 4

From St. Louis to New York and finally Helsinki, Finland. The flight from New York was 8 hours, but we made it. Been sleeping on the benches for about 4 hours! We leave for St. Petersburg in an hour. It was a little crazy flying into the sunrise and missing almost all of night time. Luckily, the plane had little TV's on everyone's seats to watch whatever you wanted the whole way!

THE HELSINKI AIRPORT WAS WHITE. Not just white, but a glossy white, like moonlight shining on freshly fallen snow kind of white. Everything from the floor to the check-in counters. If the walls weren't glossy white, they had floor to ceiling windows showcasing the beautiful views. A morning haze cascaded over the hills as the sun began to wake. Everything was spotlessly clean. The only pop of color was the bright orange seats at each terminal. I should have been sleeping like Michael, but my adrenaline was keeping me awake, and I didn't want to miss the next flight.

What are they like? What if they don't like us? What if the driver doesn't pick us up when we get there? I must smell bad! Like a dog chasing its own tail, my thoughts ran wild until it was time to board the next plane.

"And teaching them to obey everything I have commanded you, And surely I am with you always, to the very end of the age."
Matthew 28:20

LANDING IN ST. Petersburg, Russia caused a flutter of emotions. Once we stepped through the gate, we were at the mercy of whoever picked us up. We didn't speak the language, we didn't have a cell phone that worked. The butterflies in my stomach were turning to hornets.

"Well, here we go," I said to Michael.

"Is someone supposed to be here to pick us up?" he questioned.

"Supposed to be, but I don't know who or how to know."

"Do you have a number to call if they aren't here?"

I looked up at him with a wrinkled nose, "Nope." That would have been a good thing to ask for.

We passed security with passports stamped and headed out to see what awaited us. Holding hands, we looked around the very small lobby that was crowded with people. We had no idea who we were looking for, but to our surprise, there, holding our name, was a woman. We made eye contact and met her halfway. She got right to the point, not wasting a beat.

"Morgans, I am Natalia. I am to exchange money for you and take you to hotel. I arrange for plane to Kaliningrad tomorrow."

"Okay," we both nodded, not knowing what else to say. "Do you have money?" she asked.

"Oh, yes. How much do you need?" Michael started to pull out our life savings from his protective front pocket.

"Nyet, Nyet, Let's go to side. Less eyes to see," Natalia said. "I take all you have." Michael looked at me, then around the lobby, and headed to a corner. He turned toward me against the wall as he reached under his shirt to retrieve the seventy-five hundred dollars in cash we were instructed to bring. He handed her all of it; she turned and quickly walked away, across the lobby. We started to follow but decided to watch her every move.

"We could have just lost everything," Michael looked at me, rubbing his head. I couldn't even talk from the frog that was lodged between my throat and pounding heart.

Natalia stood, waiting at a small window in the wall before returning.

She quickly shuffled through the Rubles, handed Michael back a wad of it, and stuck the rest inside her coat. "Let us go," she nodded.

"What just happened?" I whispered, holding Michael's hand as we walked.

"I have no idea. She could have handed me back a hundred dollars for all I know!" As Michael spoke, I noticed the beads of sweat on his forehead. I gave his hand a squeeze. We had to trust these people.

With no real order, people and cars were everywhere. Natalia's car was parked halfway on the sidewalk, and as we drove away, she honked and waved at people to move out of the way.

The sun was shining, not a cloud in the sky. I thought, *what beautiful promises are ahead.* I couldn't wait to see what God had in store for us and decided to trust that everything was already worked out. This would be the beginning of our happily ever after.

Natalia again parked her car half on the sidewalk, arriving at the hotel for the night. She jumped out without a word and returned to the trunk of the car to retrieve our luggage, so we both got out to help.

"Everything is ready. A driver will be here to pick you up at 5:00a.m. in the morning." She walked us down a few stairs that lead to a cute, half underground, hotel room.

"Do you need anything else?" Natalia asked.

I was starving. Our last meal was on the international flight that was hours ago. "Is there a place close to eat?"

"Aaa, Da. There is pizza place just block away. So good," Natalia offered.

I smiled, "That will be perfect! Thank you so much for your help!"

"My pleasure. Remember, I send taxi at 5:00a.m., take you to airport domestic," and with that, we were all alone in a foreign country. Exhausted, hungry, and possibly broke. We decided to head out to find pizza and then hit the hay for the early wake up call.

The beautiful blue sky was slowly fading to purple, overshadowed by the towering historic city buildings. Every gray chiseled stone had been placed with strength in mind. The one-way street was narrow, barely enough room for one car, but the sidewalk was just right for two. We walked hand in hand as we turned left, smelling our way to the pizza parlor.

"There it is!" I said. The neon pizza hanging in the window gave it away.

"Glad there was a picture," Michael laughed. Down a few steps, like the hotel room, the pizza parlor was underground. Fresh bread engulfed us as we entered the dimly lit room.

"Preevyet, Padoidi syuda," the waitress said.

"English?" I smiled.

She smiled and nodded, "Oh, hello, come this way."

We exchanged a look of relief. Our first official language barrier was avoided. The waitress handed us a menu, and to our surprise, it was in English. In my heart, I felt God taking care of every situation.

"Do not be anxious about anything, but in every situation, by prayer and petition, with thanksgiving, present your request to God."
Philippians 4:6

FIVE IN THE morning came surprisingly slow. The eight hour time difference had kept us both awake for hours. Day was night and night was day, so the morning trip to the domestic airport in St. Petersburg felt like afternoon. I couldn't see it, but the sun was up somewhere, making the sky between the buildings a beautiful dusty pink.

There was no small talk with the taxi driver; that would be considered rude, and he knew where to take us. It was normal enough. With our tickets in hand, we were dropped right in the middle of the bustle of people coming and going. No one gave us a second look. We blended in with the crowd heading toward security.

Watching the other people ahead of us, we picked a line and played follow-the-leader. As friendly as any American TSA agent, the Russian security corralled us through handheld metal detectors while we wheeled luggage and backpacks behind us.

"That was it?" Michael looked around.

"I guess so. We didn't even take off our shoes." Still rolling our luggage, large cases and all, we headed toward the gates.

The crowd thinned the farther we walked. "Gates G-K," I said as we walked the halls. The gates were easily labeled. Looking down a very vacant tunnel, I said, "This must be it." We looked around and realized we were the only ones in the hall. Double checking our tickets, we decided this had to be the way, even though we were the only ones heading that way, away from the main airport.

The buzz of the half burned out fluorescent lights echoed with no sunlight to be seen. Floor lights every ten feet lit the way.

"This is large enough to drive a tank through," Michael said.

"Maybe that's what it was for!" My laugh echoed back at us.

"I bet you're right. Oh, great, a walking escalator!" Michael said.

We both headed toward the middle and noticed quickly it was not moving.

"Maybe it's too early for them to turn on." I offered an explanation, but as we continued, the floor started turning from linoleum tile to broken concrete. Yellow caution tape and orange cones blocked off the other end of the escalator. We both slowed, realizing how crazy this scene was getting.

"I hope we are going to the right place." My stomach

was in knots. I hated not knowing where I was going. "Let's walk back out and check our tickets again. We have plenty of time."

Back in the hall, a few people passed as we agreed this was indeed the way. We headed back in and continued past the broken escalator, rolling our luggage over the pieces of linoleum and concrete.

Feeling as though we had just walked a mile through the WWI trenches, there was finally sunlight at the end of the tunnel. We ascended a flight of stairs to a glass hexagon in the middle of the tarmac. Blinded by the sun, we slowly realized we had actually gone underground and back up. Benches bolted to the cracked asphalt floor rounded the structure, while a single green port-a-potty stood proudly in the middle of the large space.

"Oh, good. I need to use the bathroom," Michael said.

"You're going to use that?"

"Surely it's hooked up to something," he laughed. I was skeptical as I watched him enter and then turn right back around. "Nope, just a hole! I have to go. I'm going back out of the tunnel."

"And leave me here? Alone?" I was nervous.

"Well, yeah. It seems pretty safe here."

"What if the plane comes and you aren't back?"

"We don't leave for another hour, Samantha. It's going to be alright. Just stay with all the luggage, and I'll be right back," he assured me.

I stared across the tarmac, watching planes fly away in the distance. My sweet kids have been waiting for us. Our first meeting would be nothing short of magical. I couldn't wait to hold and comfort them. I had a backpack full of goodies that I lovingly picked out just for them. Things they might never have seen.

Michael returned, as promised, as other people also started arriving. I felt more at ease, but still wished I could ask someone where they were going. Instead, I watched. Russian people were so beautiful. Everyone was well dressed and groomed. I smiled as a mother watched her young son fly his model airplane from the seat next to her. That would be me soon.

About fifty feet away, a plane pulled up and parked; the door opened as stairs were wheeled over and attached. The crew exited and work began. A graceful stewardess walked to our glass hexagon to unlock the door, her black hair pulled back and pinned just so under her hat. The whole scene reminded me of the 1942 movie *Casablanca*; down to the age of the plane.

"How old do you think that plane is?" I looked at Michael nervously.

Michael mirrored my concern. "Good question."

We had no idea what was happening, so we waited and watched the other passengers. A cart was brought to the door, and one by one, people loaded their own luggage onto it. Michael followed suit before it was hauled away, and we watched as each bag was thrown into the belly of the plane.

Shortly after the stewardess was back, she said something in Russian. Only the mother and son went to her, so we waited. We waited until everyone was in line. When we finally handed over our tickets and passports, she smiled and said, "Welcome to Russia."

I smiled, relieved that she knew we were Americans and that we must be getting on the right plane.

CHAPTER SEVEN

S tanding just outside the gate, making everyone go around her, stood a well-dressed woman. Her sign boldly read MORGAN. With her hair pulled up in a tight bun, she was all business, so we spotted her right away. Eye contact was made and she headed straight for us like a torpedo.

"Michael and Samantha Morgan?" she asked.

"Yes!"

"Welcome to Kaliningrad! I am Tatiana, adoption agency's social worker. I will coordinate everything for you in Russian. How was flight?"

"It was a long trip, but all the flights went smoothly," Michael offered.

"Wonderful." She started walking and talking, "We must go first to Secretary of Education to accept offered children before you can meet them." Michael gave me a sideways look, and we took off after her. She walked as quickly as she talked, but she knew exactly where to pick up our luggage. "You stay tonight in Kaliningrad, and then we meet your driver and translator in the morning." By now we were informed and standing by her car.

Michael loaded the luggage in her forest green four-door Corolla, and we climbed into the back seat, buckling our seat belts.

She drove as fast as she talked and walked.

"You must be busy." Michael broke the silence.

"Oh, yes. I have three families come at same time! Your children are at Baby Home Number Two in Gusev. It is two hours away. I coordinate everyone's drivers, translators, and paperwork. A driver and translator will pick you up in the morning from hotel lobby. I have another family to get from airport!"

Buildings and signs were a blur in the car window. Michael loved history and couldn't wait to see Kaliningrad. He had done his research and was excited to experience it.

"Did you know this used to be part of Germany? They lost it after World War II." Michael was looking out the window.

"No, I didn't know that," I laughed.

"Oh, yes, Kaliningrad is beautiful," Tatiana said. "So much history. The buildings and even people are more European than the rest of Russia."

There would be little time for sightseeing this trip, but I was sure we could eventually. I knew this little piece of Russia wasn't connected to the mainland, much like

Alaska, but I only knew that from looking at a map. Kaliningrad was the largest city in this little piece of Russia, sandwiched between Poland and Lithuania. I hoped to visit the Baltic Sea while we were here.

"This part of Russia was once German. Many World War II military bases here. Still main Russian military bases are here," Tatiana shared as she drove. "Soviet Union took land from Germany after war, but now no more Soviet Union, we have President like America. President Putin so handsome." Michael and I smiled at her comment. President Putin had just been elected again for a third term, ignoring the two-term limit.

The Secretary of Education building was limestone blocks top to bottom, looking larger and more important than the rest, surrounded by grass and trees. Tatiana put the car in park and turned to face us.

"No worries here. We go in. I will talk for you. The Secretary is big man, but he is not to worry about. Everyone wants good families for our children. All you will have to answer is yes when I ask you if you would like to see these children. Da?"

"Yes, Da!" We entered with a nervous excitement, but I knew we would exit with the future just ahead of us.

At the top of the stairs was a single office no bigger than a bedroom. Standing behind the large wooden desk was an even larger man. He greeted Tatiana as they spoke in Russian; he laughed a jolly laugh and pulled a manila folder from one of the many filing cabinets against the wall.

We sat in the oversized chairs in front of his desk that Tatiana was half leaning on. He landed heavily and placed the file on the desk in front of us, saying something to Tatiana in Russian.

Tatiana looked at us and asked, "Do you wish to visit Yegor and Krishina?"

"Yes," we both answered. I smiled at the man; he smiled back and winked sweetly.

"Uspeha I moi pozdrovlenia," he spoke again to Tatiana.

"He says good luck, and congratulations," she translated.

THE DRIVE from Kaliningrad to Gusev was just over two hours of country roads and cobblestone village streets. It was a relaxing ride after the busy morning. Tatiana had other things to do and traded us off with a driver and translator. As we drove, I admired the simple country scenery that surprisingly reminded me of home. Wide open grassy fields, electric poles in the distance, but there were no billboards, and oddly, no fences. I giggled at the sight of an occasional cow grazing in the field. Without fences, the cows were tied with a chain to a large tire or sometimes a cement block.

Our driver, Domi, pointed out the large bird nests on top of the electric poles. They were made by the large white baby delivering storks. He boasted that they only built their nests in the cleanest air that lacked pollution. As a little girl, I read all the nursery rhymes about these storks who delivered babies. I watched the fields as the birds flew, and felt like I had been living a fairy tale, waiting for the happily ever after.

Gusev was a quaint little town, not a village, but small, where the Pissa and Krasnaya Rivers meet. The main road through town was two lanes, but people drove like it had three lanes. The street was lined with store fronts and people walking to and fro. It forked, and as we turned right, I could see the beautiful city center with trees, park benches, and statues of military leaders gone by. What a beautiful place for a beautiful new beginning.

Baby Home Number Two was off the beaten path. Just a block from the main street, the road turned into a mix of asphalt and dirt. The back of the orphanage came into view and couldn't be missed. An old green chain-link fence surrounded the perfectly square grounds. The building was getting a face lift with a bright shade of lime green stucco. Rounding the corner, we could see the front of the building, all three stories of it were outlined with scaffolding. The tattered and worn soviet gray remained on the front from years of communism. This place was a construction site.

We pulled in the gated property onto a dirt, pothole-filled driveway, maybe a parking lot, I couldn't tell. A manual cement mixer and other construction tools were littered about. A dilapidated shed, barely standing, rested in the back corner, but in all the chaos, I noticed the yard.

Surrounding three sides of the building was a small, colorful, well-kept playground. Dirt and spots of grass lay under old fashioned swings and monkey bars with every pole painted a different primary color. I could tell they made do with what they had, and what they had was well-loved.

A sweet little grandma met us at the car. As she spoke in Russian with our translator, Elina, I took everything in. I felt at peace, like the plan was finally coming together. It was as if God was saying, *"Get ready, this is going to be amazing."* The smell of concrete and dirt filled the air; there was nothing really nice about this place. It was surrounded by other old buildings and an overgrown vacant lot. Birds were singing, but other than construction and birds, it was eerily quiet.

"Isn't this place full of kids? Where is the laughter, or even cries?" I whispered to Michael.

The translator turned around, smiling, "Inga, the director, says we have to climb up the fire escape to get inside. Are you okay with that?"

With wide eyes and raised brows, I glanced at Michael. I shrugged and said, "Okay, yeah. We can do that."

The fire escape would have had a hard time passing code in America, but it would do. From the top, I could see the whole town. Hundred-year-old buildings lined the cityscape. German in design, but many ruined with a coat of soviet gray stucco. To the right, the city turned into country, fields dotted with little shacks and dirt roads.

After snapping a few pictures, I turned and ducked

through a window, following the rest of the group. My feet hit the floor of a closet filled with coats, clothes, and supplies. The group headed out the door, and I was surprised to be in a large room surrounded by small children ranging from two to five years old. Some were eating lunch at a child-size table, while six, maybe seven, were lined up against the wall, pants pulled down, sitting on small training potties.

"Eat, restroom, nap," Inga said in broken English, pointing to where those took place, obviously proud of the structure and schedule of her orphanage. Again, I found it odd to be in a room full of children with very little noise. The children looked clean enough and cared for, but there was something lacking. The other side of the room was lined with toddler beds and cribs where a few children were already napping. Overwhelmed by my surroundings, I forgot to even look for Yegor and Krishina. They could have been here, or maybe there were more rooms just like this.

Down a few flights of crumbling concrete stairs and through a small nondescript wooden door, we stepped into another world, immediately transported into a beautiful lobby entryway. The ceiling had to be three stories high. Stained glass flowed, selecting only the green light to shine in. We followed Inga up three flights of beautiful, ornate wooden staircases to enter a spacious office.

Three rows of heavy, unused wooden chairs sat in front of bookcases and filing cabinets like soldiers. A flimsy, compressed wood, L-shaped desk surrounded

Inga's secretary with stacks of paperwork piled on all sides of her. She was young and petite; her straight brown hair fell to her shoulders as she smiled.

We entered another office, clearly Inga's. Everything was old. Bookshelves covered two walls, connected in the corner by a black velvet chair where Elina sat. We were seated opposite of her, on the matching velvet couch closer to Inga's desk. As Inga talked, I couldn't help but gaze out the only window behind her. I couldn't see anything but clouds, but at least the clouds were familiar, as I found myself lost in the Russian language.

Inga retrieved a file from the rows of filing cabinets and took her seat behind her desk; she spoke in Russian, but Elina translated, "Michael, do not be upset if the children do not like you. They do not see men. Only man that come are to fix plumbing or heating. So they may have never seen a man."

Inga told us about our kids, how long they had been with her, and medical information. Mostly the same information we knew before coming.

"Samantha, Michael, we come back to meet the kids. It is nap time right now," Elina said.

"Oh, okay," we said, a little shocked at having to wait, but there was nothing we could do. It was mid-afternoon, I would rather them be rested.

"You come back today at 3:00p.m. You will visit every morning 10:00a.m. to noon and every afternoon 3:00p.m. to 5:00p.m. Da?" Elina stated.

"Da." I smiled at Inga. She stood and nodded,

motioning us to the door. We scaled the fire escape and climbed back into the car to grab a bite to eat. Elina took us to a quaint little bistro with floor to ceiling windows. A free Wi-Fi sign hung by the entrance and I was also able to update our family and friends.

September 5

Eating a late lunch, or early dinner, waiting to see the kids! Met with the Secretary of Education this morning then traveled 2 hours to the orphanage. Met the orphanage director, and now we wait to meet the kids until 3:00. (8:00a.m. your time). :) Will let you know more later!

CHAPTER EIGHT

The lime green orphanage shined like a beacon calling us back. Each step felt like a step closer to motherhood. We entered up the same rickety fire escape and arrived in the first office with rows of wooden chairs.

The secretary motioned for us to sit and then turned to leave. On the edge of my seat, my mind never stopped. *What will the kids be like? Will they like us? Will they cry? What should I do when I see them?* A million questions ran through my mind. A million what-ifs were about to be answered, and I just knew it would all be better when I got to hold my kids.

Moments later, a busty nurse dressed in white from head to toe held little Yegor's hand and edged him ahead, followed by the secretary carrying Krishina on her hip.

I was taken back a moment at the sight of Yegor. He was missing the front two inches of hair down to his scalp. His hair was already so thin and malnourished. He looked like a little old man who had lost his hair. It had either fallen out or been shaved down to his scalp.

Clinging to the leg of the nurse for safety, he didn't dare make eye contact. The tears began as the secretary handed me Krishina and went to her seat behind the desk. Krishina was so tiny, my carry-on luggage weighed more than her little frame. I smiled and tried to comfort her. Michael stayed back, hoping to ease the situation while the nurse pried Yegor off her leg. She exited the room, closing the door behind her.

I bounced Krishina while holding a hand toward Yegor, who was banging on the door to escape. So much for the glorious union I had envisioned. Krishina wouldn't let me hold her too close. She hung loose on my hip, leaning as far away as she could as I tried again to coax Yegor away from the door. Looking at Michael for something, anything, I knew he couldn't help. I was at a loss and couldn't even speak their language.

"They hate me!" I began to cry.

"Samantha, they don't know us."

"Easy for you to say, they told you they would hate you. Kids love me. They were supposed to love me," I said.

The secretary spoke to Yegor in Russian. It sounded stern, but the Russian language did. He was still hiding behind the desk looking suspiciously around the corner, but at least he had stopped screaming and banging. Krishina kept her eyes on her brother, but she had also stopped crying.

"Okay, okay. You're right. It's going to be okay," I said

out loud, as much for myself as for the kids. The secretary couldn't speak English, but I knew she was watching. *Jesus, give me strength.* After my little prayer, I remembered my backpack full of toys and books. Holding Krishina, I plopped down on the floor and scooted my backpack close. With wide eyes and raised eyebrows, I gave Yegor a mischievous grin. I looked between Krishina and Yegor as I slowly unzipped the pack, looking inside only to close it quickly. With a curious smile toward the pack, I opened it again only to stick my head in and back out with excitement. I knew I couldn't speak to them, but a smile, a laugh, facial expressions are universal.

He didn't look away this time, obviously intrigued, but he didn't give himself up that easily. I opened the backpack and slowly pulled out a toy car. Yegor's eyes lit up, but still he kept his distance. I laid it on the red ornate rug and pushed it in his direction. Next, I pulled out a little teddy bear for Krishina. Then another car and some puzzles.

Krishina's tears dried up quickly and her curiosity about this amazing backpack took over. She nearly fell in head first. As Krishina played, Yegor watched. She sat on my lap to read a book while Yegor listened. Inch by inch, he moved close enough to pick up the toy car. Moving closer still until he was within arm's length. I made no effort to reach for him, instead I reached in the backpack and pulled out a teddy bear for him too. He smiled, grabbed the bear and took a step back again. At four years old, he had been hurt more than Krishina. He could possibly remember the day they were left here. My heart hurt for him. *Lord, what have these babies had to endure in their short life?*

He was dressed in cute red overalls and a white and red striped tee shirt. Blue and pink socks showed from the tennis shoe sandals velcroed on his feet. Krishina was swallowed whole by a pink and blue striped dress with an oversized red sweatshirt thrown on top to match her brother. The workers had tried so hard to dress them in matching outfits. Pink tights covered in large blue hearts and finished with red sandals. They were taken care of, definitely not abused or mistreated. Like the playground outside, the workers here didn't have much, but they took care of and made the best of what they did have. Although very outdated, the children's clothes were clean and mended.

The question in the back of my mind was still there. *Have they been loved? Could these children bond with us if they didn't know what it was like to love or be loved?*

Krishina began to play. Her little smile emerged slowly, and she even handed a few toys to Michael. We all found common ground. Finally, I removed the board books from the pack and sat crisscross on the floor in the middle of the room. Yegor came, took a book from my hand, turned and plopped down in my lap. I breathed a sigh of relief. As I held him, he jabbered and pointed at the pictures in the book. Krishina was all over the place, not walking as good as a two-year-old should, but still enjoying the new toys that she didn't have to share.

Michael was observing quietly, knowing it may take longer for them to warm up to him, but Krishina jumped into his lap giggling. We looked at each other with huge smiles, both realizing we could fall in love with these kids and finally have a family.

After about two hours with the children, the same nurse came to get them.

"Da, Deti idiemte." She must have told the kids to clean up because they quickly put everything back in the backpack. I encouraged them to keep the bears, but the worker would not allow it. After cleaning up, Yegor and Krishina left with little emotion. They didn't even look back.

"For I am the Lord, your God, who takes hold of your right
hand and says to you,
Do not fear; I will help you.'"
Isaiah 41:13

SLEEP WAS CALLING OUR NAMES. It was so late by the time we arrived back to Kaliningrad. Tatiana had already taken us to dinner and dropped us off for the night. The MockBa Hotel was historic on the main street of Kaliningrad. It was beautiful. The red carpet led us upstairs to our room. Not much different from any American hotel, except the electrical outlets, but the beds were amazing, so we felt right at home.

It didn't matter what time it was. It was time for sleep, because all was well in my world. Breakfast would be available in the hotel restaurant in the morning and then off to Gusev to see our kids again. We both melted under the covers and drifted away.

"I will say to the north, 'Give them up!'
and to the south, 'Do not hold them back.'
Bring my sons from afar and my daughters
from the ends of the earth."
Isaiah 43:6

CHAPTER NINE

"Would you like to stay in Gusev or Kaliningrad?" Tatiana asked. I didn't even have to ask Michael. "I'd rather stay in Gusev than make that drive every day!" I said.

"That will make easier for me, and you can visit longer. Let me talk with Elina and then you go. There are two hotels in town," Tatiana said, and I took the chance to update the family.

September 6

We are eating breakfast now, then head out again to the city they are in. We're going to get a hotel there so we can walk to the orphanage. I hope they don't cry this morning when they bring them in! Here is a picture from yesterday.

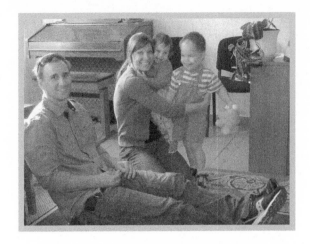

BECAUSE OF THE DRIVE, we would have a quick visit this morning before finding a hotel. We climbed the fire escape again and followed the same path to the office. Like before, the secretary left and returned with the same nurse and our beautiful children. This time they recognized us, or should I say, they recognized the backpack. There were no tears this time, but they were cautious. Krishina's smile warmed my heart.

"They remember us....and the backpack!" I laughed.

Much like yesterday, we played, became comfortable with each other, and truly started to bond. Yegor was even warming up to Michael. Michael bounced Yegor on his knee, and Yegor showed him all the animals in the books. They really played. Yegor fell in love with a tub of small animals I had brought; lining them up on the chair one by one. He especially loved the giraffe.

His hair was slowly growing back, and I was able to ask why it was shaved.

"Shave for rash, ointment on head." The worker's English was so broken, but she understood I was concerned about his hair. Although, I wasn't sure if she was telling the truth. I knew with proper nutrition they both would be healthier and with a forever mom and dad, they would be happier too. We learned that no relatives had come to visit them in two years; even with an aunt in the next town over. I was told that was somewhat normal when the family couldn't financially support extra kids; they would bring them to the orphanage.

"May the God of hope fill you with all joy and peace
as you trust in him, so that you may overflow
with hope by the power of the Holy Spirit."
Romans 15:13

"WE NEED to find hotel and you can walk back in afternoon," Elina said. We parked directly off the square and watched Elina go in. She came right back out. "They say they have no room, but I know they do. They do not want to give to Americans."

"Because they don't like us?" I asked.

"No, because they do not think they have nice enough room for you."

We pulled down an alley and parked on a dirt lot behind an unmarked building. I knew why she tried the other place first. This looked a little shady.

"I'll be back, see if they have room." Elina got out and went in the back door.

"This is a hotel?" I looked at Michael. His shoulders raised and lowered in disbelief.

Elina came back to the car, nodding her head. "Da, they have a room. I had to talk them into taking you. Owner do not speak English. It is closest hotel to orphanage, and she has breakfast each morning in restaurant downstairs. You can walk down the street and turn left on corner with grocery store to orphanage."

We climbed out of the car and started unloading suitcases, careful not to place them in a mud puddle. We followed Elina in and up a narrow staircase just wide enough for the largest suitcase. The hall had only a handful of doors to choose from. She walked to the end of the hall and unlocked the door with a large gold key, stepped out of the way, and waved us into the room.

"Is this fine here?" Elina asked.

"Oh, yes, this is just fine." I didn't care what it looked like.

"Then I will go now, and Domi will pick you up at orphanage noon on Friday. There is nice bistro on square where we ate yesterday."

She nodded and was out the door. After the door was

closed, I took a deep breath and released the most emotional two days of my life.

I turned in the narrow hallway, not much wider than my own shoulders, to peek at the small bathroom that fit a shower, toilet, and pedestal sink. The hall opened to a room no wider than seven feet. My college dorm room was bigger than this. This would be our shoe box for the next five days. Yellow, possibly indoor/outdoor carpet grounded the two twin beds that lay catty-corner to each other in the room and only a foot between them. Michael had already claimed his bed under the one small window.

KNOCK KNOCK KNOCK, someone at the door startled us.

"Preevyet," I answered.

An older woman with a furrowed brow and cordless phone in her hand looked me up and down. She pointed to the phone, "Da, Da," and handed it over.

"Hello?"

"Hello, I am granddaughter. My grandmother does not speak English. She needs your passports to report you stay with her." The young girl spoke English well.

"Okay, we can do that. Just a minute." I handed the phone back to the woman, smiled, and pointed one finger in the air for her to wait. I retrieved the passports and handed them over. The woman smiled and nodded her head in approval.

"Spasibo," she said. I was picking up enough Russian to know that was thank you, and of course, 'da' means yes, and 'nyet' means no. I would have to work on learning more this week.

"I hope she brings those back," Michael said. I was too trusting. I hadn't even thought about her not returning them.

"Well, was there another option?" Not needing a reply, "We have enough time to find food. Are you hungry?" I asked.

"Yes, starving!" Michael sat up from bed.

The cute little bistro with huge windows overlooking the square was just what we needed. We ordered whatever we could find on the menu with a picture and enjoyed our time together. I had brought my computer, seeing a free Wi-Fi sign last time. Our hotel room had Wi-Fi, but it was not the best. I wrote to our family, knowing they would be waiting for much more information than I had been giving them.

September 6

We visited again. Yegor's hair is growing back. They said he was getting a rash or something, so they shaved that part to put medicine on it! I think I would have shaved it all. They remembered us, no tears this time! We were able to stay in a hotel in the same town, so our interpreter, Elina, and driver, Domi, left us for the next few days.

We are close enough to walk to the orphanage, and we can visit twice a day in between nap time. Ordering dinner last night was fun! They couldn't believe Michael wanted plain water with no fizz in it. I stuck with the safe Koka Kola!

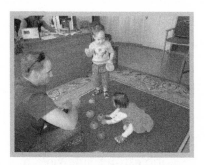

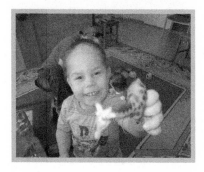

I ADDED pictures from the past few days, and then we headed back to our shoebox to rest. *Thank you, Jesus, for this gift. Protect my babies and make them their favorite!*

We had time to take a quick nap until knocking woke us up. Answering the door, I was greeted by the little babushka, looking much happier than before.

"Spasibo," I said, smiling ear to ear as our passports were returned just in time to head to the orphanage. Collecting things for my magical backpack, I looked around our small room. It was already a mess; we had unpacked and dug in every suitcase. Packages of crackers and snacks were thrown on the bed to make room for toys in the backpack. Michael had washed some clothes in the shower and hung them to dry on the window. I wasn't too worried; we would get it all put back together soon. The messy room could wait. I was ready to see my kids. We closed and locked the deadbolt with the heavy gold key and headed for our kids.

Walking the cobblestone sidewalk to the end of the block, we turned left and walked until the sidewalk turned to dirt. This would be our normal for the next four days.

***

OUR STROLL home that afternoon was precious; we held hands like we were dating again. It was nice to just be us without the worry and stress of work or what was happening with the adoption.

"Should we keep their Russian names as middle names?" I asked.

"I think that is only right, don't you?" Michael said. "I think it would be impossible and cruel to just start calling them by a new name at this age," he added. "So, Maverick Yegor and Reagan Krishina?"

I smiled, "Yes, Maverick and Reagan!"

"I like it, I think those names fit them, although I may just call Yegor, The Tank," he laughed.

As we passed the grocery store on the corner, we noticed a few baby strollers lined up.

"Well, I guess that's stroller parking," I laughed, but as we got closer, it became clear it was more than that.

"Michael, there is a baby in that one, and that one!" We looked around and saw no one. The babies were swaddled, some sleeping peacefully, but my goodness, how dangerous. In America, someone would snatch that baby up. It was so different there, like stepping back in time.

Life was hard. Everyone did what they had to survive. Selling produce on the side of the road, sweeping city streets with a broomstick; no job was overlooked or beneath them.

Reflecting on the past few days, my heart was heavy for the people here, and our kids. What kind of life have they lived so far? The trauma they must have from being abandoned. Especially Yegor, he was old enough to remember. We would never have known this world existed.

We were exhausted, but by 9:00 p.m. the sun was just setting and sleep was nowhere in sight. I knew our family and friends would be waking soon in Missouri, so I used the time to watch the videos we took of our kids, decide what pictures I liked best, and post to the group.

September 6

We are staying in the city of Gusev for the next few days.

I don't even know what to say, except we are ready to bring our kids home...It's midnight here, I better get to bed! Good night!

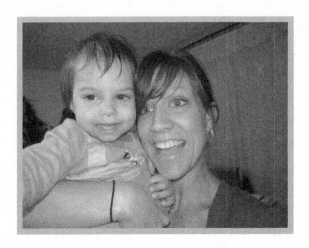

OUR BODIES WERE SO confused by the time change, sleep was so messed up. It was hard to fall asleep and stay asleep. I was up again much earlier than I wanted to be.

The next few days played out much the same. We would spend the whole morning together until it was time for lunch and naps, then we would return for a small visit each afternoon. By afternoon on the third day, the sky was getting dark. We waited in our hotel room as long as we could.

We donned our jackets and prepared for a wet walk. I brought new toys, and Yegor was especially thrilled. Orange and green sunglasses in the shape of stars were first, and he wore them with pride, although he soon decided he liked Michael's better. We played with everything until all we had left were bubbles. They had never seen such amazing things. With their little eyes as big as saucers, Michael blew the first few. In Inga's office, we had some privacy. He didn't go crazy, just a few were enough. The kids jumped and giggled, popping the bubbles. Krishina crawled all over Michael for the bubble wand. Before we knew it, our time was up and we had to say goodbye.

Although the kids enjoyed our visits there was still no emotional connection for them. They were neither excited to see us or sad to go, but each time we said goodbye they took a piece of my heart with them.

GUSEV WAS A BEAUTIFUL LITTLE TOWN. The weather cleared to blue skies, so we strolled away from the familiar path to the orphanage and headed toward the square. A picturesque cobblestone bridge arched over the river that ran through town.

To the right of the bridge was a quaint park bench, adorned on each side with a sculpture of twisted iron rooted from the ground to form the trunk of a tree. Branches and leaves tangled the top. They would have looked just like a tree had there not been padlocks covering them both. All different shapes, sizes, and colors of padlocks. Several were red in the shape of a heart.

"What in the world is that?" Michael laughed.

"How funny to padlock a tree. They're cute, let's take a picture with them!" As we sat closer I noticed more, "Most of them are engraved with names and dates."

We continued over the bridge to the square that was surrounded by huge evergreens. They were so huge you couldn't see what was inside without going in to explore. Michael was soaking up the history, knowing much of WWII was fought nearby. In the center of the square was a statue of some military leader gone by. It was refreshing to be outside in the sunshine. With the cover of the evergreens, I felt free. No one was watching our every move. No one was babysitting us. This just felt normal.

Returning to the hotel, I Googled the padlock tree for something to do. "Aw, Michael, the tree is a symbol of love. When a couple gets married, they attach a padlock to the tree and throw the key in the river to symbolize their strong lasting love."

Michael huffed, "Well, there ya go."

"Oh, don't be such a cynic. I think it's sweet. We could bring a lock when we take the kids home and attach it for our family!"

"Whatever you want, honey," Michael teased, but he meant it. He flew around the world this far, and we might as well attach a lock to a tree if I wanted.

I posted pictures from the past few days and then went back to watching film of my precious babies.

September 7

We walked a little in Gusev today. This is a marriage tree. People getting married put a lock on the tree to symbolize a strong marriage and throw the key in the river! The bigger the lock, the stronger the marriage! Cute idea.

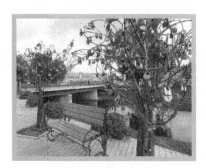

"WHAT DO you think it will be like taking them home?" I asked Michael.

"I think Yegor will be a handful!" he said.

"Yeah, the language will be a problem for a little while," I agreed. Michael covered his face to finish his nap. I closed my eyes to rest but didn't sleep. I was dreaming of my kids and the future.

WHEN WE ARRIVED on the fourth day, we were taken back outside to the playground. We waited on a small wooden bench inside a little lean-to with three walls. It was a nice but brisk September morning. I was glad for the new freedom and loved that they trusted us to be alone with the kids.

The young secretary and a nurse escorted the children out, but once Yegor saw us, he left them behind. This is what I had been dreaming of. It took longer than I expected, but it felt so much better than I could have dreamed. He was truly excited to see us. With my arms opened wide, I swept him off his feet. I noticed the little secretary covered her heart with her hands. His small gesture had not only melted my heart, but hers as well.

Krishina, bright and happy, was placed in Michael's arms. So much had changed this week. The children were both truly happy to see us, and I knew we could bond even more once we were home.

This beautiful morning had a crisp chill in the air. We had already taken off our jackets, but the children were bundled up like it was below freezing, adorned with coats, hats, and boots. The best part of their wardrobe was the little plastic sunglasses we had brought them yesterday. The workers actually let them keep them, and Yegor wore them with pride, pointing and showing me right away. He was ready to play, and I could tell he had been here before and knew right where the bikes were.

"I think he's glad he doesn't have to fight the other kids for the bikes!" I laughed, "and he looks like a happier little boy with the stocking cap on."

"Yeah, well, it covers up his missing hair!" Michael laughed.

"Oh, you're right! That's what it is!"

We played and laughed for over an hour. It was so nice to feel more like a normal family, instead of being watched in a small office. Up and down the sidewalk, Yegor shuffled his feet to make the bike go.

"He looks like Fred Flintstone!" We laughed. "Maybe he doesn't know how to use the pedals?"

Michael ran after Yegor as I held Krishina's tiny hand. She was turning two in October, but wasn't walking well enough on the uneven grounds to trust her completely. I scooped her up and placed her in an oversized wooden baby swing. Her giggles brought me so much joy knowing she was finally warming up to me.

Inga stopped by to say hello, but I knew her real motive. She didn't look happy about the kids being outside. She spoke to them in Russian and felt their hands to see if they were cold. I couldn't help but smile at the loving care Inga gave each child here. I could tell they were loved and cared for. Just as she smiled and started to leave, Yegor tried to take a little bicycle from Krishina, causing a fight.

"Nyet, Nyet Yegor," Inga said. She smiled, pointing a finger in the air. "You learn nyet, no, quick!" She laughed and waved goodbye.

We smiled and agreed. I took Yegor to the swings distracting him from the conflict. We played and laughed, but the favorite by far were the bubbles! I soaked up every moment, knowing tomorrow would be our last and shortest visit before leaving the kids until October.

We hugged them goodbye and kissed each cheek. As they walked away, Yegor looked back and waved. That little wave said so much.

———————

MICHAEL TURNED the key to our little hotel room and entered slowly with a gasp.

"What, what is it?" I was pushing past to see a completely spotless room. There were no shirts hanging to dry, no dirty clothes piled anywhere, no computer laying on the bed where I had left it.

"We've been robbed!" I said. Michael was still looking around in shock.

"If we've been robbed, why are the beds made, and where's all the trash?" he noticed.

"Well, I don't even see my suitcase!" I started investigating, opening the dresser drawers. "Oh, thank God, here is the computer and my Bible and journals." Opening the closet, I found my suitcase with clothes hung and folded neatly in piles.

"We didn't get robbed, they came and cleaned!" My neck and face went flush as I realized this had to have taken much longer than they needed to spend on one room. "Oh my gosh. This place was a disaster; I am so embarrassed!"

September 8

We get one more short visit this afternoon with a social worker there. We are still not sure if she will be watching us or wanting to talk to us.

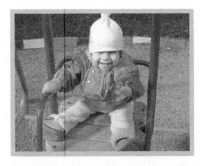

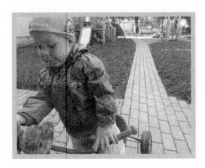

I POSTED to the family before leaving. Dragging all of our luggage behind us on the cobblestone sidewalk, we walked slowly, knowing this would be our final day. Stroller parking was empty at the grocery store, no babies waiting today.

Michael spoke up, "So what's next? After today, I mean."

"Well, we get picked up at the orphanage today and then we catch our flight to Saint Petersburg tonight at ten. We have a whole day there with nothing planned. The next day we finish our medical exams and fly home."

"But we have most of our medicals done, right?" Michael left all the details to me.

"Yeah, I gave them to Tatiana when we got here."

"Good, that's the last thing I want to do is anything in a Russian hospital."

"We should just have a physical. Then Tatiana will have to let us know when we come back for court. She said we could be picking them up by Christmas!"

We walked on, talking about the kids. Laughing about Maverick Yegor's hair and Reagan Krishina's spunky personality.

Content--that was what I was feeling, content.

"Hope deferred makes the heart sick,
but a longing fulfilled is a tree of life."
Proverbs 13:12

"Can we get a family picture before we have to go?" I asked.

"Da, Da." The workers were there to take the kids. I just wanted one last photo of them as a family. We stood and gave the camera to the worker. Reagan Krishina in Michael's arms and Maverick Yegor, The Tank, as we had lovingly nicknamed him, in mine.

I talked and shifted him every which way to try to get him to smile at the camera, but he was not having it.

The nurses were all making noises and faces, talking to him in Russian. The nurse spoke to the translator. "She says it is nap time."

Something on the shelf had his attention. I spotted a black pony and grabbed it for him. He grinned and admired the pony like a treasure.

They snapped the last family picture with the little black pony so proudly part of this new family. As the kids walked away with no emotion, I waved my last goodbye.

"I'll be back soon," I said. Neither one had an emotional connection to us yet, but soon we would be a family of four.

"And we know that in all things God works for the good of those who love him, who have been called according to his purpose."
Romans 8:28

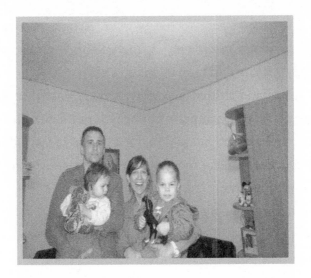

CHAPTER TEN

Time spent in Kaliningrad was a whirlwind, and just as fast as those five days went by, we were already in St. Petersburg to finish the medical evaluations.

"The cardboard sign with our name must be for us," I laughed. It was crazy how trusting and comfortable we had become traveling. I hadn't worried as much about who would pick us up. Our agency had been spectacular so far.

We climbed into the driver's car and away we went into the night. Like from a postcard, Russian landmarks came and went. I did my best to take pictures of scenery, even in the dark. The Mariinsky Ballet, The Bronze Horseman, other monuments and architecture we didn't recognize; there was so much we were missing in the dark. It was well past 2:00a.m. by the time we arrived at the same hotel. With nothing planned but sightseeing tomorrow, we crashed on the beds without an alarm set and fell fast asleep.

WHEN I FINALLY WOKE FROM hunger, a sliver of sun poked through the curtains. Checking the time, I knew exactly what I wanted for lunch. Pizza. We didn't have any plans for the day, so we showered and got ready for the little pizza parlor. It was a beautiful, clear day and would be perfect for sightseeing.

"Let's walk to the end of the street after lunch and see where it leads," I offered. I woke with so much hope for the future; I couldn't sit still all day.

"Okay, but I'm not walking too far!"

"Oh, hush, how often will you be in St. Petersburg?"

"But I have flat feet!" Michael insisted. After lunch we stopped by the room, where I grabbed my backpack as we headed back out the door. We learned quickly that Russians didn't baby anybody. If you wanted something, you had to do it yourself. No one would be checking on us to make sure we were sightseeing, or even eating, for that matter.

A casual stroll up the road led to some beautiful architecture that drew us in. The city was breathtaking and busy with activity. Our hotel was conveniently placed within walking distance from St. Isaac's square, a popular tourist destination. Beautiful, not a cloud in the sky, I breathed in the moment and barely touched the cobblestone sidewalk. As if out of a painting, an arched brick bridge led over a small man-made canal. Just ahead, the golden dome of St. Isaac's Cathedral. It towered over the garden park with each detailed sculpture carefully placed to tell a story.

The park was bustling with people, and we didn't seem out of place with all the other tourists enjoying the sights. The Monument to Nicholas I towered overhead, taking up the center of the park. A wedding party in the grassy gardens to our right were taking pictures. The bride and groom's laughter was contagious. I couldn't help but smile the whole time. Even Michael, with his flat feet, was in awe of the history.

"Do you realize the oldest buildings in America are only around 300 years old?" he asked.

"SO..."

"These buildings are at least twice as old," he educated me.

Laughing and enjoying our free time, we had walked miles from our hotel when we noticed storm clouds forming over the Baltic Sea. This beautiful day had quickly turned gray and cloudy, but nothing could dampen our spirits. Out of instinct, I packed away the camera and we started back to the hotel.

Huge rain drops started to fall, one by one, followed by a downpour. Within minutes, the water came down in sheets and there was nowhere for us to hide. We ran as far back as the arched bridge when I stopped. A giggle bubbled up in my throat as I laughed out loud, "We are miles from our room, where are we running to?"

"I don't know," Michael laughed.

Who would have ever guessed we would be in St. Petersburg, Russia, caught in a rain storm about to become parents by adoption? We stopped to find ourselves in the middle of the canal bridge, laughing and smiling at our predicament. Just as the century-old buildings lined the canal that led all the way to the Baltic Sea, I felt bigger things were in store for us too.

The sadness of infertility brought us to this point, but how could we be mad about that? We laughed and walked in the rain together and I heard that small voice once again, *"I alone can bring happiness from your storm, trust me."*

"Now faith is confidence in what we hope
For and assurance about what we do not see."
Hebrews 11:1

MORNING CAME QUICKLY. It was dark, but the hospital was a busy place. Medical evaluations would be quick, I had already given what was done in the United States to Tatiana. We entered the building with two other couples also adopting and were directed to an old-fashioned coat check, like in a 1950s movie. We gave the woman our coats and received attractive paper booties to slip over our shoes. It was clean and, although dated, looked similar to a normal hospital.

The group waited in a somewhat normal waiting area before being called in, one couple at a time. Finally, we entered and sat in front of a huge wooden ornate desk. It seemed everyone important had a huge wooden ornate desk.

"Hello. Michael and Samantha, Da?" she said.

"Da, Preevyet," I said.

"Da, you have medical files completed?"

I looked at Michael shocked, "Um, yes. We gave those to our agency worker, Tatiana, in Kaliningrad."

Now the woman looked shocked. "We need here."

"Well, we don't have them. She took them from us as soon as we got there. She never said we needed them here."

"Oh, never give medical information to anyone. It is private." The woman looked concerned.

Never give medical information away, I thought. *Why not? We have been handing over thousands of dollars to strangers since we got here. Who cares if someone has an X-ray of my lungs?* Someone must have turned the heat on, I started to sweat. How could this have happened? I looked at Michael for support, but he was just as clueless. Surely they could mail or fax them.

"Here, have tea. I call Tatiana." I didn't really want the tea, but when in Russia, you drink tea. So I took the cup and sipped it slowly. Even though the Russian language sounds like an angry language, the woman's tone was quite compassionate. She hung up the phone and smiled a sad smile.

"She says she have them, but did not know you give both copies to her. I'm sorry, but we can do them here. Not a problem. Da, never give medical away!" She reminded us again.

"Redo them? All of them? They can't mail you what we have done?" My heart sank to the floor. Michael and I both hated needles, and I definitely didn't want to do any of that here. I saw Michael lower his head, and I knew exactly what he was thinking. We would have to redo the TB test, X-rays, EKG, blood work…… Tears began again, I couldn't be strong any longer.

"Nyet, I am sorry. We need them today for adoption."

I was a whipped puppy slumped in the wood and leather chair. My skin went cold and a nervous clammy sweat began to form.

"If that's what we have to do, we will," Michael offered.

Leaning forward, I placed my head in my hands and cried. How could I have been so careless? I knew Michael would be upset. I had let him down, and I didn't want to do this either. This was the last hurdle to jump, and I face-planted.

"Dear, you okay?" the woman asked. I gathered myself and sat up. Wiping the tears and pity party away, I said, "Yes, I'll be fine."

"It will be good. We will take good care of you," she said, patting my back with sympathy.

We were whisked away with the other couples down the hall and into a stairwell that was cold, falling apart, and reeking of smoke. Crumbling concrete pieces ripped at the blue paper booties covering our shoes.

"What's the point of these booties?" Michael jokingly asked. I wasn't ready to laugh yet, but observed the irony of them. I gave a halfway grin, looking straight forward and nodding. With a side hug and a smile he said, "It's going to be alright." I nodded, but looking up at him made me start to cry again.

Back inside the hospital walls, the nurse split the men and women. She wore a white nurse's gown that buttoned up the front with a white cap adorned with a red cross on the front. It was classic 1950s nurses wear, down to the white shoes and panty hose.

"Women first. Follow me."

I left Michael behind to enter a large room with a huge circular contraption in the middle—which, again, looked like it was also from the 50s--that was supposed to x-ray our lungs.

"Shirts off."

We all looked at each other. There were no hospital gowns offered, none lying around to put on.

"Shirts and brazier off. Line here." The nurse pointed to a bench against the wall. My face turned three shades of red as I looked at the other women.

"Seriously?" Again we looked at each other until one offered to go first.

"Da, shirts and brazier," the nurse said again, clearly

put off that we were not ready yet. The three of us stood, covering ourselves with our arms, waiting in line to step into the x-ray machine. I lowered my head into my hands that were so conveniently curled up by my head, hiding like a toddler. Maybe if I couldn't see them, they couldn't see me.

One by one, we stepped into the machine. Like being held at gunpoint, I was told to hold up my hands as the contraption circled around me, x-raying my chest.

I didn't talk; I just wanted all of this to be over. We were returned to the hall as the men were escorted in. After they had their turn, we headed on to the next chosen torture, although I didn't think it could get more embarrassing.

"Oh man, we've got to do the blood work again." Michael turned white.

Feeling so guilty and on the verge of tears, all I could do was squeeze his hand and say, "And a TB test. I'm so sorry. This is my fault."

"I didn't mean it like that; it'll be okay!" he wrapped his arms around me as we waited. We were the last couple to draw blood; Michael decided to go first. I didn't like needles either, but I could get through it. As he exited I asked, "You alright?"

"I'm good, the nurse was actually awesome," he replied. I smiled and breathed easier knowing he was finished with that. I sat, looked away, and kept my eyes closed the whole time. I felt the nurse rub and pat my arm in comfort. I only nodded in appreciation, and before I knew it, I was finished as well. I joined Michael and the other couples as we headed to the final exam.

"This should only be a physical, so the hard stuff should be over." I offered the information only because I needed the comfort myself.

Up a few flights of stairs, we were led to benches in a quiet part of the hospital. After the first couple exited, I grabbed the woman's attention.

"What's next? You guys were in there a while!" I asked.

"Psychological evaluation. She just asked questions," the woman offered.

I nodded and thanked her. I forgot about the psychological evaluation we had paid hundreds of dollars for back home, reminding myself how much time and money I had wasted with this one simple mistake.

We sat together in front of a pleasant, smiling young woman, not at all what I was expecting. She asked about our marriage and why we were adopting. She asked about our infertility struggles and if it had caused any marital problems. She asked about our extended family, jobs, likes and dislikes, favorite hobbies and interests.

I thought this was the most enjoyable part of the morning, by far. We left her office, and I felt relieved it was almost over and the only thing left now was a routine physical.

Again, I was the last to finish. I entered the sterile exam room with a medical table on one side and a blank white plaster wall on the other. There were three nurses in the room with charts and equipment. All seemed normal until I stepped on the scale to be weighed and measured. A door I had thought was a closet opened, and in walked another nurse who walked through like the room was a hallway. The other nurses ignored her and continued on.

I took my seat on the exam table as they took my temperature and checked my reflexes. All normal stuff until, "Take off shirt and brazier, pozhaluysta," a nurse said matter-of-factly.

"Me, why?" I asked, pointing to myself as if there were anyone else they could have been talking to.

"Da, off." The nurse motioned upward with little care as to what I thought. I waited a moment, expecting one of them to lock the doors, but no. So here I found myself, taking my shirt and bra off again in a room I just saw someone walk through like a hallway.

"Down," the nurse said, pushing my shoulder toward the table. I laid there, feeling exposed and vulnerable, praying no one else would walk through that door. I stared up at the ceiling as they used a stethoscope to listen to my lungs and take my blood pressure. The nurses wheeled over a cart with the oldest EKG machine ever created. Black tubes ran from the machine to little suction cups as they got to work suctioning them to my chest. I closed my eyes, wishing them away and praying for invisibility, although I knew I had to endure it. I kept my eyes closed as I heard the door open and close, open and close. The Russian language filtered in and out of my mind.

If I kept my eyes closed, no one else existed. I could

listen to the hum of the machine and think of my kids, forgetting what was happening at the moment.

Finally, they started removing the suction cups. I opened my eyes to see a nurse smile and say, "Almost done. Breast exam."

Great, let's top this off with a breast exam! I closed my eyes again to head back to my happy place as the nurse did her job. I was shocked back to reality when the nurse pinched my nipples. My eyes opened to them writing on the chart and speaking in Russian. I didn't know if they were making fun of me, as if that was a joke. They didn't say anything to me, but I could tell they were finished, so I put my shirt and bra back on as quickly as I could.

As I joined Michael in the real hallway, he looked at me with knowing eyes.

"You alright?" he asked.

"No, I have never been more humiliated in my life!" I whispered under my breath. "I can't imagine ever having anything more embarrassing than what just happened to me."

Michael's eyes were wide and curious. "That bad, huh?"

"You have no idea! I just had a breast exam in a hallway, complete with a nipple pinch," I said.

"That's not normal?"

"NO, that's not normal!" I didn't want to talk. I was on the verge of tears and couldn't help but feel guilty at what had transpired this morning. It was all preventable.

We retrieved our coats from the check-in counter and

threw away the ripped up booties. I couldn't wait to get to the hotel to pack our bags and go home.

SEPTEMBER 9,

I am so sick of Russia! I want to go HOME!!!!!!! Medical evaluations this morning in St. Pete were the most stressful thing I have ever done in my life!!!

I COULDN'T EVEN EXPLAIN to the family how terrible the medicals really were. Thank God that part was over, but flying into New York City on the tenth anniversary of September 11th might trump that.

We touched down at JFK to make the trip from international to the domestic terminals, only to be met with hordes of people. Every shape, size, color, and nationality, only God could have imagined. Two distinct lines formed; UNITED STATE CITIZENS or NONCITIZENS. We read the signs and thought we were in the correct line, but we didn't feel like we were. This small-town girl was overwhelmed, but as always, I tried to put on a brave face. Everyone who looked and talked like us was in the other line, and no one in the citizen line was even speaking English. Another fork in the road had us choosing another path; CLAIM ITEMS THIS WAY.

"That sign says to claim any items like food, grains,

nuts..." I read, looking at the bag of nuts in Michael's hand that he wouldn't throw away on the plane.

"Well, I have these." The small bag of nuts from Helsinki began to feel like a problem. The large Indian family in front of us looked to have an entire house worth of belongings boxed up on three carts that nearly hit the ceiling. As we stood and waited, we noticed customs officers were going through everything.

"Are we going to have to wait for them to unbox this house in front of us?" I said, "I knew security would be tight today, but we are not going to make our next flight if we wait here. Maybe you can throw those nuts in the trash."

"Yeah, I don't think this is what they meant by claiming items," Michael agreed, but by now, we were committed. The man with the house was ignoring us, and downright rude as we asked a security guard what to do.

"We don't have anything to claim." I said to the guard, "we thought these nuts from the last airport counted."

"You no try cut. No cut!" The man in line interrupted, pointing a finger at us, as we now ignored him, looking as clueless as we actually were.

"Oh, you kids come on this side then, and throw those nuts away right there," the security guard said. "Thank you so much," we said as she lifted the fabric fence and we dragged all of our luggage, never looking back at the man. Everywhere we went, we were met with kindness, even down to the TSA agents.

Past customs, JFK was a city in itself. We took the

airport subway to the domestic terminals, where we waited again in a huge security line. We were becoming pros at removing our shoes and following orders like cattle. After two more security checkpoints and swimming through people, we made it with just a moment to catch our breath.

"Let's avoid JFK next time," Michael suggested.

"Yeah, this was crazy. I think we can fly internationally from Chicago," I said.

CHAPTER ELEVEN

I wasn't shy about our adoption, it's not like we could hide it. I posted publicly to Facebook and shared our new family and the kids' beautiful faces. I was so proud. My profile picture included my kids, but I kept the personal stuff for our private page. We had a month before flying back for our court date and visiting our kids again. Having them home before Thanksgiving would be sooner than I had planned! Working with our travel agent, we decided to make two more trips. The next for court and the last to bring our kids home. The option was discussed to stay in Russia between trips, but living there for four weeks wasn't an option with work.

SEPTEMBER 13,

We just found out we will have to make 2 more trips...If

we stay the whole time, it would be 4 weeks in Russia. We still leave the 17th of October, but fly home after court on the 26th. We will fly back for the kids around November 13 to be home with them around the 16th.

IN THE MIDDLE of expanding our family, we also moved into our new home. There wasn't much to clean, so like any nesting mother, I was busy preparing the nursery with a coat of gender neutral green on the walls. The light wood crib would be perfect for Reagan Krishina's bed, and we still had time to find a small twin bed for Maverick Yegor. I brushed my hand across the bright colored circles on the bedding. It would be perfect for both kids, as I was preparing to add pops of pink and orange for the shared room.

We had plenty of room now, but keeping the kids together was important to me. This wasn't just a big change for me and Michael; it would be a life-changing event for Yegor and Krishina as well. I just wanted it to be as smooth as possible for them. They were about to lose everything and everyone they had grown to know the past two years, and be thrown into an unknown world with unknown people. My pain and loss from infertility came first for us in this journey to build a family, but my children had also endured the trauma of losing their biological family. Coming home with us would take familiar people, a familiar home, along with losing their culture and language.

These scars would always be with us. Although scarred in different ways, I hoped our love would be a healing ointment for us all.

I continued to work, painting picture frames I had gathered; pink for Reagan and orange for Maverick. My adorable children would soon be framed and hung on the wall. I received my grandmother's old rocking chair that fit nicely in the corner with a large R and M hanging above. A perfect room to start a new chapter in everyone's life.

THE WHOLE SCHOOL district was so excited for us. After years of keeping the secret of infertility, it was like the flood gates had opened. We couldn't keep our adoption plans a secret, and we didn't want to. As I drove to the elementary school for a baby shower, I was overjoyed at the reality that this was really happening. It didn't feel real.

I entered the gym in awe at the amount of people who were there. I searched the crowd, making eye contact with everyone I could. I couldn't hold back the tears. Happy tears from years of waiting. This baby shower would be a rite of passage and another step closer to motherhood.

I found my dear friend Jamie, who had also waited so long to become a mother, and we hugged and cried. We were part of a different kind of club. A club no one wants to be in, but once you're there, you have each other's back; because infertility changes a person.

"It's your turn now," Jamie said. I could only smile at the outpouring of love from everyone. "Come, sit down over here!"

"Thank you, oh my gosh. This is too much!" I sat down as I spied the mountain of gifts, the huge cake, and the sea of people. There were smiles all around, and each one felt a part of our story.

They brought me gift after gift to open. Boy clothes, girl clothes, shoes, toys, and of course, books. Everyone had signed my favorite gift so far, titled "God Found Us You" by Lisa Tawn Bergren.

I read the sweet words of Little Fox asking about the day he came home. The day it made his mama the happiest mama in the world. I imagined my kids asking me those same questions one day.

I cried. It was impossible to hold it in. Soon I would be just like Mama Fox, finally bringing my babies home. One by one my coworkers, and my friends, came to congratulate me with hugs and excitement.

This is what it feels like to be expecting, I thought.

The rest of the month flew by with more showers, gifts, paperwork, and travel plans. I watched the videos of Yegor and Krishina every night, and I even made a video of our trip. I updated our family and friends on the group page.

September 16

Okay...didn't want the whole world knowing when we would be gone from our house! Our court date is set for Oct 24th. We will have to fly back out October 17th or 18th. We have to be there five days before court and a ten day waiting period after court. So we will fly home between court and Gotcha Day. Then two days in Moscow with the kids to change names and birth certificates and get passports.

OUR NEXT TRIP was so close. Maverick and Reagan's new clothes were washed and hung with care. I had even picked out the perfect outfits for Gotcha Day, although that was still a trip away.

"What should we get them for Christmas this year, Michael?" I giggled at the idea. I already knew what I wanted for them, but it was fun talking about it.

"You really shouldn't go overboard this Christmas, you know? They could be overwhelmed." Michael was always the practical one.

"Well, don't you think they need bicycles? That's not overboard, is it?" I made a face. Michael laughed, knowing he had little control over this department. I had dreamed of this moment for years; seven years, to be exact. I was justified in going just a smidge overboard if I wanted.

CHAPTER TWELVE

My phone rang during school, a little unusual, but I looked anyway. It read 'ADOPTION ASSOCIATES AGENCY.' We were leaving in two days for our court date, maybe there was a change in travel plans. My students knew we were adopting, they would understand. I pushed the answer button quietly.

"Hello."

"Samantha?"

"Yes, what's going on?"

"I have some news, is Michael with you?" Our case worker Oksana sounded concerned.

"No, I'm at school right now."

"Can you be with him soon? I think we need to talk about this together."

"IS EVERYTHING OKAY?" I couldn't stand this guessing game.

"Let's talk about it with Michael there."

"Okay. Let me get to a place I can call him, and I'll call you back."

"That's fine, I'll be waiting."

It was halfway through the school day when I hung up. I was in the middle of 5th period, but the students were working on an assignment. I stepped next door and asked Mrs. Watson to watch my class so I could make the call.

The office buzzed like a bee hive with students coming and going. It was a busy place, but the secretary knew right away something was wrong. "Are you okay, Sam?"

"I'm not sure yet, I need to call our adoption agency," I said.

The principal was standing there as I halfway asked, halfway helped myself to his office. When I stepped inside and closed the door, every scenario was filling my head, each one worse than the one before. *Court may have been delayed, or travel details needed changed. Maverick must have gotten hurt on the playground. Maybe Reagan was sick; maybe they were both sick. What if the orphanage caught on fire?* My breathing labored and my palms were sweating as I called Michael on the school line and told him about the call. I put him on speaker and dialed the agency from my cell.

"Adoption Associates, this is Oksana,"

"Hello, this is Samantha and Michael, we are both on the phone."

"Thank you for calling so quickly, are you together?"

"Yes, I have Michael on speakerphone."

"I think you will need his support."

"Will you please just tell us what is happening?"

"You are sitting down, yes?" Oksana questioned.

"YES!" I sat down on the edge of the nearest chair.

"Da, okay. The aunt of Yegor and Krishina was contacted about they being adopted to America. All families must be notified before they can be adopted. This never happen, but the aunt wants the children, I am so sorry," Oksana finished.

The aunt wants the children. "I'm sorry. What do you mean she wants the children?"

"Yegor and Krishina's aunt want to take custody of them to raise. She wants them, and you cannot adopt them." When Oksana spoke those words, I crumpled to the floor. My dream had just died at that moment. Unable to speak, my phone hit the floor.

"She knew for years they were in the orphanage!" Michael said.

"Yes, it is unfortunate. There is new law in Russia encouraging families to keep Russian children in Russia. The aunt will more likely get paid to keep them."

"So she wants them for the money?" Michael asked. Even over the phone, Michael knew I couldn't finish this conversation. He knew I was broken, not just heartbroken, but my spirit was broken.

"I'm afraid so. Samantha, are you alright?" Oksana asked.

"What's next, what do we do now?" Michael asked.

"Unfortunately, we do not have other children for you right now, but you must still appear in court to stop the adoption of Yegor and Krishina."

"And if we try to fight for them?"

"That is not even an option. Aunt is Russian. She will win because she has priority over you. Your best option is to stop adoption so you can move forward with other children. Samantha?"

"Okay, so we fly to Russia, appear in court, and hope a child becomes available while we are there?" Michael said.

"That will be plan for now. I call you if I hear anything further," she offered.

"Thank you, Oksana," Michael finished.

"Michael, please see your wife. Tell her I am so sorry. Samantha, darling, if you listening, we will have other children. Do not be worried."

I hung up. The white concrete walls were closing in on me. I had to leave. I knew everyone outside the door could hear me crying. They all knew it wasn't good news by now. The linoleum tile underneath me wasn't cold enough. I rested my head on the chair to pray, but all I could cry out was, "Why?" I collected myself enough to get up. Sitting in the chair, my phone rang again. This time it was Michael, but I didn't want to talk.

I collected myself enough to ask to leave for the rest of the day. I couldn't answer, "Are you okay?", "What happened?" questions over and over. I didn't even know how to answer them, let alone teach.

On autopilot, I collected my purse as quickly as possible, walked down the long, white hallway, and slammed the metal door open as hard as I could.

"No temptation has overtaken you except what is common to mankind. And God is faithful; he will not let you be tempted beyond what you can bear. But when you are tempted, he will also provide a way out so that you can endure it."
1 Corinthians 10:13

EVERYWHERE I LOOKED WAS A REMINDER. My car already had a car seat and a booster seat for my kids. I only had a couple of miles to drive home, but with every turn I became angrier. *This isn't fair, GOD! Why? That aunt has never wanted them, or even visited them, for the past two years! WHY?* I pulled into the garage where the empty boxes were piled from nursery items bought or received.

I slammed the door and headed straight for the nursery. The nursery that I had so lovingly prepared for my children. The nursery that my children would never see. In the middle of that perfectly painted, pea green room, I dropped to my knees. My blood pressure was boiling over. I looked around with blurry eyes and grabbed the closest thing I could reach.

Freshly painted pink and orange picture frames that hadn't been hung yet. I threw them with everything in me, and they shattered on the wall, just like my dreams. I pulled out the dresser drawers, grabbing handfuls of little socks and underwear, pants and tights that had been washed and put away. I tore the bedding from the bed. As I stood at the closet, I grasped each little outfit, imagining how fast Maverick would have run or how graceful Reagan would have twirled for her daddy. I hated the thoughts and began tearing them off the hangers as well.

In the middle of this war-torn room, on top of the debris, I curled up in a fetal position and wept.

They were MY babies. Mine! Not a soul could hear my cries, my wordless groans, but even through the pain I felt His words in my heart.

"No, daughter, they are mine. 'But if we hope for what we do not yet have, we wait for it patiently."

This is not what I want. God, why? I told them I would be back. But I felt nothing in return. Only warm tears running down my cheeks.

"Samantha? Where are you?" Michael yelled through the house. Time had stood still. I don't know how long I had laid there. It was only by the comfort from God I had fallen asleep.

Michael entered my broken world in disbelief. He looked around the destroyed room until his warm eyes met mine. I raised my arms in surrender. My broken and fragile heart needed to be held together.

"Do you feel better?" Michael asked. I could only shrug my shoulders like a pouting toddler. "This won't bring them back," he said while stroking my hair. I nodded into his shoulder, knowing he was right. Nothing could be done, and we laid on the floor together and cried.

"In the same way, the Spirit helps us in our weakness. We do not know what we ought to pray for, but the Spirit himself intercedes for us with groans that words cannot express. And he who searches our hearts knows the mind of the Spirit, because the Spirit intercedes for the saints in accordance with God's will."
Romans 8:26-27

CHAPTER THIRTEEN

As Michael parked the car to make the long trip yet again, my heart ached. It was late morning, but my feet dragged behind and the bags under my eyes puffed from the lack of sleep for two nights. In my fit of rage, I had deleted all evidence of Yegor and Krishina on Facebook, both public and private. The news would have to spread the old-fashioned way, because I didn't want anyone's advice or sugar-coated words. I was in a dark place, a place I would never want to admit. Was this really God's plan, or had I just taken the idea and ran with it? I even asked myself if there even was a God, though I never spoke the words out loud.

Are you there, God? What are you doing to me? You must have me confused with someone stronger, someone more capable. You aren't supposed to give me more than I can handle!

As we were walking in the parking lot, my phone rang.

"It's the agency." I handed the phone to Michael with a halfway eye roll.

"Hello, this is Michael." I anticipated the worst as he listened intently. "Okay, so she is almost a year and a half?" Michael glanced my way. "Okay. Thank you, I'll let Samantha know."

"They have a little girl we can see," he said, hanging up the phone.

"Hmm," I grunted, keeping my gaze forward.

"Samantha, that's good. I know it's not what you envisioned, but she needs a home too."

Now I could add selfishness to the long list of emotions I felt today. "I know that, and I'm a terrible person for feeling this way." I paused, not knowing if what I had to say should be said. "I feel like we are going to the pound to pick out a new puppy." There, it was out. Tears started again. "This is not how it's supposed to happen!" I said.

"Maybe not, but it is what's happening. You have to hold it together. We'll know more when we get there. Yegor and Krishina have a family to live with."

Michael tried consoling me, but he was pretty much dragging me through airport security. I envisioned our oldest being a boy, but then again, maybe God didn't give me that vision either.

"In my distress I called to the Lord;

I cried to my God for help.
From his temple He heard my voice;
My cry came before Him, into his ears."
Psalm 18:6

SEAT 24B. I quickly sat down to prepare for the first of many flights. Watching the other passengers, I wondered where they were heading. Some dressed in business attire, looking bored at the whole process; others looked casual, possibly taking a fun trip somewhere nice. I wondered if they could see the cloud of hurt and disappointment surrounding me. I tried putting on makeup this morning, but my eyes were still puffy and swollen. A mother and child walked past as I lowered my head.

Lord, I can't do this. This is too much. Where are you? Why would you send me Yegor and Krishina just to take them away? I don't understand. I thought this was what we were supposed to do. Not really a prayer, but more of a conversation. Prayer was for the good Christian. The Christian who had everything under control. The Christian that only had to give thanks. I used to be that Christian, but not anymore. I was on the bad list for some reason.

Before we left on this dreaded trip, I went to see Joy to find some understanding and comfort. She had given me a card and instructions not to open it until I was on the way. I leaned back in the chair, took a deep breath, and opened the card as I dried the corner of my eye with my sleeve.

Despair walks away thinking God doesn't care.
Faith waits, knowing that in God's perfect time He will speak.
His delays are always for a reason.
He can be trusted. He is faithful.
Your life is in God's hands - and that's the very best place to be.

"Dear Samantha,

I know this has been a difficult journey. You've been waiting, hoping, and praying for a very long time. Please know you are not forgotten, and you are never alone! As we surrender to God's plan and His timetable, amazing things happen. You and Michael are in our thoughts and prayers.

'There's a miracle in the making
One just for you, the Father is working even now
Your prayers have been heard
And the answer's on the way
There's a miracle in the making for you today!'

Much love, Joy"

Joy's friendship and guidance had meant so much over the years. I read the card three more times before putting it away. As I settled in the seat, my heart heard a sweet whisper from Romans, and I gave way to sleep.

"I consider that our present sufferings are not worth comparing with the glory that will be revealed in us."
Romans 8:18

"WHAT DO YOU MEAN DELAYED?" I asked.

"I'm sorry ma'am, they are having trouble getting the tow off the plane. They should have it off any minute," the stewardess explained.

Stranded in the Chicago airport, I was already on edge, and a delayed plane couldn't have come at a worse time. We had a very short layover in Germany. I knew every minute we waited would affect the rest of this trip.

"Relax, hon, we will leave when we leave," Michael said, as he put his feet up. He was never one to panic, especially when he doesn't know what's at stake.

"How can I relax when our layover in Germany is less than two hours? Do you know what that means? We are going to miss our connecting flight. That will also make us miss our domestic flight in St. Pete if they don't get that tow off!" Heat grew red-hot up my neck. I paced the windows, staring at the passing planes. Michael knew to just let me stew, there was nothing he could do at that point.

"Everything about this trip is wrong, just wrong," I said.

Finally, after an hour and a half of pacing, the plane pulled into the gate. Maybe, just maybe, we would have time to make the connecting flight in Frankfurt.

WE WERE the first out of our seats, and had prepared to have everything ready to go when the plane touched down. After the nine hour flight from Chicago we let the stewardess know our situation. She was so kind and updated us as we grew closer. She even announced for the other passengers to stay seated to allow us off the plane first. As soon as the unbuckle sign flashed, we were up and scooting down the aisle.

Like out of a movie, we were running past other travelers, pushing our way through the crowds. I thought I was in great shape, but the added backpack and stress weighed me down as I ran. My heart was burning, not just from running, but from fear. We were cutting it close, but I thought we still had a chance.

"Hurry, Michael, it leaves in 20 minutes!"

Finally we saw the check-in counter, and the plane through the window. "We are here for flight 1054 to St. Petersburg."

"I'm sorry, that flight has already been loaded. I'm afraid you are too late," the attendant said.

"No, NO WE CAN'T BE, it's right there; I see it! Our last flight was delayed."

"Miss, please."

"WE RAN ALL THE WAY HERE, I SEE the plane, IT'S RIGHT THERE!" I was starting to draw attention.

"Miss, I'm sorry, the walkway was removed twenty minutes ago, we have been calling your name," she said with no compassion.

"Our other flight was delayed! Can't you reattach the walkway?" I said, but she was starting to get annoyed.

"No, we cannot." Throwing my hands in the air, I turned and slid down the counter with a frustrated cry, curled up in a heap of backpacks, tears, and sweat.

"Why is this happening? How much worse could this trip get?" I said aloud. I knew full well the flight attendant and people watching were thinking, "Spoiled Americans," but I didn't care. This was the worst day of my life--no, the worst week of my life. This entire situation was spiraling out of control. Losing the kids, a delayed plane, missing connecting flights in a foreign country. What else was going to go wrong?

Michael finished the conversation with the attendant, as I finished my tantrum on the floor.

"Get up, you look ridiculous!" Michael pulled me off the floor.

"I don't care," I huffed.

He pulled me in tight, releasing hours of frustration. I

usually had it all together. I could usually calmly think three steps ahead in emergency situations. Thank God for Michael. He was there to pick up the pieces when I most needed it. Surrounded by his hug, a deep inhale was released and I regained my composure.

Nothing could be done. All the events leading up to this point were out of our control. I knew I had to let them go.

"We have to find a computer or Wi-Fi so I can get a hold of the travel agent. Then I have to contact the agency and let them know we are stuck in Germany!"

"Is not God in the heights of heaven?
And see how lofty are the highest stars!"
Job 22:12

WE FINALLY ARRIVED BACK at our familiar hotel room in St. Petersburg. Not a planned overnight stay, but at least it was familiar. I updated the family on Facebook.

OCTOBER 20

Well, we have made it as far as St. Pete tonight. The plane in Chicago was delayed 2 hours due to not being able to get the tow off the plane. We only had 1 hour 45 min to catch the connection in Frankfurt, Germany...missed it by less than 20 minutes after running a mile in an airport with backpacks on. Rebooked on a flight that left almost 7 hours later. (Yes, we sat in Germany for 7 HOURS; well, ran for some of that.) That made us miss the domestic flight we had booked tonight. So....a great start to an already great trip! We are staying the night in St. Pete tonight and fly out at 7:00a.m. We'll see what happens tomorrow.

CHAPTER FOURTEEN

Tatiana picked us up from the airport just in time for court Friday morning. I never knew soviet gray was a feeling. It was a sad feeling, devoid of any future or hope. Everything, even the sky, had a fog of gray as heavy and gray as my heart. Today would be hard.

Lord, I don't know where you are. Please, if you are listening, please hold me up today. Have mercy on us. I didn't know what else to pray for. Maybe it was insulting to question where God was, but why hide what was in my heart.

I wondered if there was a dress code for court, but jeans would have to do. We sat waiting on the hard wooden benches for what felt like an eternity. The two-toned, eggshell, great grandma-esk wallpaper was a stark contrast to the dark wood of every stick of furniture in the courtroom. The room was longer than it was wide, and along the left wall were clearly cages for the criminals.

Two large boxes constructed of wood and plexiglass looked oddly similar to a dunk tank at a carnival. In front of those were possibly the defendant's tables. Instead of facing the judge, they were straight across from the prosecuting table. Grounding the whole scene in the front of the room was the judge's massive perch, much like someone would see in America. There was no room for a jury. By the looks of the cages, a criminal was clearly not innocent until proven guilty. The only spot of color was the bright red Russian flag.

Finally, our translator, Elina, came back. "They are ready to start and will be in soon. There is no need to worry." She sat next to us with no more small talk. As promised, just a few minutes later, in walked the judge. Brows furrowed and dressed in an oversized black robe with a large white ruffle tie hanging down from her neck, she walked straight to her podium. The parade following behind her consisted of the orphanage director, Inga, her secretary, a lawyer or two, Tatiana, and possibly another secretary.

Stern and serious, as with everything, the judge rapped her gavel, her oversized wooden chair swallowing her small frame, but she spoke with confidence. Mesmerized by the language and exhausted by stress, the conversation drifted past my ears. Everyone was quite serious, I couldn't tell if it was because of the circumstance or the Russian culture, but I couldn't help but get the feeling this court appearance was different and even unusual. Everyone's eyes stayed glued on us, yet avoiding eye contact.

The look of pity was universal and transcended language. I thought, *Maybe this doesn't happen often and they are truly upset for us and the children.*

"Samantha, what do you say?" Elina's voice rattled me awake. "Do you wish to stop the adoption of Yegor and Krishina to move forward with other children?"

Shaking from head to toe, I took a deep breath. Michael had already answered; they were all staring at me.

I squeezed Michael's hand and answered, "Yes." The finality of the situation overtook me. My dreams for Yegor and Krishina were dead; as if they were dead. Our future was so uncertain, I began to cry. I tried to do all the things to stop while I looked up to heaven.

The judge spoke kindly in broken English, "We are truly sorry for loss of children. This does never happen. We agree how deep you care for children." With a choking, tight throat and blurry vision, I forced a grin and nodded in agreement. With sad smiles all around, court was adjourned.

"Be strong and courageous. Do not be afraid or terrified because
of them, for the Lord your God goes with you;
He will never leave you nor forsake you"
Deuteronomy 31:6

THE ORPHANAGE DIRECTOR was no bigger than the children she cared for. Her petite frame drowned in her clothing, yet she carried a sweet grandmother quality. She motioned for us and Elina, walking closer to huddle with only the four of us. I leaned down to listen. Even though I didn't understand a word that was said, I was certain it was to apologize again, so I just nodded and smiled.

When she finished the translator said, "Inga says she picked out a baby for you. She feels terrible for what happened, so she picked out baby for you." Inga was watching me for a reaction. She was smiling and nodding her head in approval.

"Pohoji na, Papa," Inga said.

"She says, looks just like dad."

"Come, come now, da," Inga said. She reached down for my hand to squeeze.

"She wants you to come today."

My mouth fell open and my eyebrows questioned. "Really?" I was still in shock and overcome by the moment.

"Da, mal'chik. Come." Smiling, sweet Inga patted my hands, smiled again and walked away. I didn't know what to think.

"Yes, a boy," the translator repeated Inga's words. I breathed in God's goodness.

"The Lord will fight for you;

you need only to be still."
Exodus 14:14

WE SLID into the backseat of Tatiana's car, still wondering what had just happened.

"Well, I was going to surprise you, but I see Inga already told. She has baby boy she picked out for you. He is only ten months old. This is very rare for Americans to get such a baby! Inga felt terrible for what happened and wanted to make the situation better," Tatiana said smiling.

"Now, we go to Secretary of Child Welfare to request seeing more children. He will offer you girl that you already know about. You will not act as you know about this boy. Do you understand? He must not know you know about the boy."

"Yes, we understand!" we both said in unison, not really surprised. This was Russia after all, everything felt a little under the table.

"He will offer you both children because you have applied for two. If you want both children, you have both. We will go to visit boy today because Inga is waiting for us. She wants you to meet him today and girl tomorrow, she is in different orphanage farther away."

I couldn't help but smile at God's work and feel guilty for fighting him the whole way. I had questioned Him every step of the way. I wondered where He was. Maybe, just maybe, we were finally about to meet our son and daughter.

Lord, I'm so sorry. Thank you for your forgiving grace. Please keep Yegor and Krishina in your arms. Protect them as they grow, bless their aunt. I pray she loves them like her own. Lord, you know they will always have a piece of my heart. Whatever your plan is, here I am. I am yours.

I felt in my heart God had this planned from the start. I can't know or understand what God has for Yegor and Krishina's future, but I know He loves them. They are His children. He has plans for them as well.

"But he said to me, 'My grace is sufficient for you,
for my power is made perfect in weakness.'
Therefore I will boast all the more gladly about
my weaknesses, so that Christ's power may rest on me."
2 Corinthians 12:9

CHAPTER FIFTEEN

The two-hour drive to Gusev was mostly in silence. I was lost in my own thoughts. We hadn't even seen a picture or medical information, but it just felt right. God himself orchestrated this meeting. I let myself dream of who he was, what he looked like, why he was here. *Would he like us? Would he be healthy?*

"Are you okay Sam?" Michael asked.

"I am, I'm just overwhelmed." I paused for a moment, "I'm excited, but also nervous that this boy and girl are only five months apart. It would be a lot like having twins. I'm worried that they aren't siblings, and I'm still worried about Yegor and Krishina."

"There are a lot of what-ifs and things we can't control," he said.

"I know, but I can't keep my mind from wanting to prepare for what's to come, or not come."

Michael squeezed my hand and without a word I knew he understood. Nothing else needed to be said.

IT WAS THE SAME ORPHANAGE, the same office, the same secretary, but this time was different. Not only were we able to use the front door, but this baby boy had been handpicked for us. I truly didn't know whether to laugh or cry. The day had been a rainbow of emotions. It's not every day one goes from complete loss and unknown, to surprising joy and possibly designed destiny.

We sat on the same couch as before, my heart racing and my leg bouncing to keep up. I stood, pacing the floor, wanting to be in the perfect place when he came in. Michael was ready with the video camera, when in walked a worker dressed in white. Time slowed as she carried this most precious little bundle of joy. My joy. My son.

I stood anticipating, with my empty arms aching for this moment. He was perfect, big brown eyes, soft brown hair, and those ears! Ears that were much too big for his little head, but oh so cute! The worker placed him in my arms, and I melted. His soft bottom lip pouted as one single alligator tear started to fall. He didn't know me, but he soon would.

"Shh, Mama's here, Mama's here. Shh it's okay." I wrapped my arms around him, and we bounced and swayed to my words, words I had waited years to say. I couldn't help but cry right along with him, but my tears were tears of joy and sadness. Sadness that he was about to lose everything he had known for the first year of his life, and joy that we were both about to gain a family.

He wore a soft, baby blue footed sleeper with a smiling polar bear fishing for a red fish. He was small but filled in the outfit just right. I could tell they had just washed him and put on the cleanest, nicest clothes they had. Inga stood immediately and said, "His name, Nikita. It means unconquered, very strong masculine."

"Nikita, don't cry. Shh. Don't cry, Nikita. It's okay, Mama's here. Shh. Don't cry." I used the back of my finger to gently wipe away his tear. Bouncing him in my arms, I breathed in his sweet baby smell. This was even better than I had imagined. We stood there for what seemed like only a minute, but things were happening around us. People were walking in and out speaking in Russian, Michael was videoing, but for me, time had stood still.

"Now to him who is able to do immeasurably more than all we ask or imagine, according to his power that is at work within us."
Ephesians 3:20

MICHAEL WASN'T WATCHING the baby. I could feel his gaze fixed on me. He knew what this moment meant. He knew the pain that had been endured to get to this point. If we lost this baby like the last kids, he might lose me in the process. The years of infertility wasn't easy on our marriage, more accurately, I hadn't been the same person he married. I had been bent past the point of breaking and longed to be truly fulfilled. Yet, he loved me through the hardest times and held me together when I was broken.

"What do you think?" Michael asked.

"Michael, he's perfect! He really looks like my brothers, as odd as that sounds."

Michael handed me a rattle we had brought, and I sat us on the floor to play, still having to support little Nikita. Even at ten months old, he wasn't fully sitting up by himself. I freed his tiny feet from the tight shoes that were over the one piece sleeper. Michael gathered a few toys from the shelves and sat them around us. Nikita wasn't interested in any of them; he held tight to the toy keys as he studied me.

"What do you think?" I asked him the same question.

He smirked, "Does it matter what I think?"

"Ha, ha, ha, yes, it does matter. What are you thinking?" I asked again.

"Well, I know you see a little boy right now, but he's going to make critical decisions in our life one day. I mean, he could put us in a nursing home someday. He may have to decide to pull the plug on my life support."

"Wow, that's a lot to put on him." I laughed.

"Well, it's true. I mean, I'm happy, I'm ready. I see that having children will add another layer to life, but I always think of the future." Michael said.

Whatever the future would hold, we would do it together, as a family. I was soaking up every moment, I wasn't thinking about the future. Our family from this point on would be totally different. All of us would be together through good and bad. We would grow old together.

Nikita's little bottom lip began to quiver, his brow furrowed, and again he was unsure of the situation. I scooped him back up and placed him on my lap. He was already getting more comfortable with my closeness. My heart was full to bursting. More comfortable than before, he gripped my finger so tightly. His trust was with me now, and I never wanted him to let go.

"Michael, look at his big hands."

"He does have big hands, and big ears to go with them!" he chuckled. "He reminds me of a little old man."

"Oh, a cute little old man!" I said, clearly already the mama bear.

"How well can he move?" Michael asked.

Standing him directly in front of me, he needed my support. His little legs were so weak from the lack of attention. He looked around at the floor, deciding he would rather sit.

I placed the rattle a little ways away and put him on his

tummy. Not fast, but carefully. He inched forward on his belly, reaching hard for the toy. Unsure of what medical problems were ahead, I couldn't deny the sparkle of life in his big brown eyes.

"Now you are the one being mean," Michael said.

"I just wanted to see if he could crawl."

"Does he seem healthy?"

"He is definitely behind developmentally, but that's to be expected. To be honest, whatever health problems could be ahead, I don't care. This is it. He's our son," I said.

Michael smiled with a sweet sense of knowing my heart. The complexity and randomness of this situation could only have been orchestrated by God. He had provided, but He wasn't finished; there was another child to meet tomorrow. God had been working this situation out the whole time.

"For I know the plans I have for you, declares the Lord,
plans to prosper you and not to harm you,
plans to give you hope and a future."
Jeremiah 29:11

SLEEP CAME EASILY. So many hours of flight time, missed departures, hours of layovers, court, meeting our son for the first time, and finally the adrenaline that had kept us going without sleep for well over 24 hours had run out. The true definition of exhaustion; international adoption. I had one more task before rest would come. I had to update our family.

The devastation of losing Yegor and Krishina was all over Facebook. Everyone was very supportive, but it was hard to make the post about losing them. In my heated anger that followed the phone call, I had deleted every picture posted about our kids, publicly and in the private group. But now, our family and close friends would be waiting for an update. The last they knew, Michael and I were waiting in St. Petersburg. I knew my mother would need to know we were safe. I gathered my thoughts from the day and wrote,

---

OCTOBER 21

Court this morning. We had to sign a stoppage on our adoption application for Yegor and Krishina. The aunt will be taking guardianship of them, they said if we fight it we would lose, and it would keep us from meeting other children. So that chapter is closed. Sometimes God steps in for reasons we may never know. Without us going through that, the aunt never would have come for them.

I BEGAN to write about Nikita but stopped. No, I would hold him as close to my heart as I could for now. We still had a big day tomorrow. I finished my post.

Love you all, and we will update you when we know more.

"He heals the brokenhearted and binds up their wounds."
Psalm 147:3

CHAPTER SIXTEEN

I was so much in love with Nikita and could not help but wonder what else God had planned. We had a little girl to visit and a very big decision to make. I couldn't imagine life without Nikita at this point, so today would really decide if we would bring both children home or only Nikita.

Poised and elegant, Tatiana reminded me of an early Audrey Hepburn. As she entered the hotel lobby, I noticed her dark blonde hair, always pulled up in a bun. She was all business, all the time, although I'm sure Saturday morning was her usual day off. What a rewarding but demanding job to unite families every day. This trip would be longer with the orphanage located on the border of Lithuania. We stood to meet her as she looked around to spot us.

"Good morning, my dad is driver today. He waits

outside, I have paperwork to take at another orphanage on the way. We go?"

I smiled, "Da."

Out the door we went, and there next to his older, but well loved, gold BMW was a jolly man, much like Santa Claus if he had more hair and a beard. I could tell he was excited for something different today.

"Preevyet." I offered a Russian hello.

"Da, Preevyet." He opened the back door for us, and we melted into the leather seats. Seatbelts were quickly needed as he gunned into the busy traffic.

Soon we were off the busy city streets, rounding the country roads. We passed a man next to a bridge with a net full of fish held toward the road. A little bit later, a woman sat on an upturned bucket with vegetables lined up on the ground before her.

"What are these people doing?" Michael asked.

"Selling things," Tatiana said. "People in country have to sell or trade what they have grown or caught, like fish and vegetables, to survive. Very, um, how you say, more money in city."

I kept my eyes out the window. This was true poverty, Americans have no idea. We had no idea the depth of poverty. The car ride was quiet. I was thinking and processing all that had happened yesterday and the possibilities ahead. How quickly my outlook had changed when I truly saw God at work. Nikita was no accident; I was certain of that. I will always miss what could have been with Yegor and Krishina, but I knew they would finally be out of the orphanage.

About two hours into the trip, we slowed at a little village, not big enough to call a town. A few run down, two-story stucco buildings lined the cobblestone main street that took a hard ninety-degree turn. Tatiana's dad pulled into the mud-filled front lawn of a very old, faded yellow building. The main concrete steps led up to a large, weathered, wooden blue door. Evenly spaced windows covered the first and second stories.

"I take paperwork inside. Do you need restroom?" Tatiana asked.

"Yes, thank you," Michael said. Almost instantly as he exited the car, little heads began to appear in the windows. Children began opening windows to get a better view, as if begging for someone to take them home. My heart sank because I knew the likelihood of them getting out of the orphanage was slim. All eyes were on our car and the adults following Tatiana inside.

As I sat in the car waiting, I looked at each little face hanging out the windows. This was the reality of humanity hitting me in the face. If we had never stopped, it would have never existed in my mind. So much of the world goes on without anyone knowing the cruel reality. *Why God? Why allow this to happen?*

Michael and Tatiana's dad returned before her.

"This is the saddest thing I have ever seen, these poor kids." I looked at Michael.

"It's terrible. Did you see all the kids in the windows? This is just another reason to take both kids. How can we leave one here?" Michael said. I had nothing to add to that. He was right.

"I have told you these things, so that in me
you may have peace. In this world you will have trouble.
But take heart! I have overcome the world."
John 17:23

THE DRIVEWAY WAS long and bumpy, but I could tell this orphanage was different. The building was aged, yet beautiful. Light blue stucco with dark navy trim. It was quaint, like out of a fairy tale, surrounded by nothing but trees on one side and a river on the other. We never noticed driving through a town, but we must have been on the outskirts of one.

"Wait here. I have to get someone to come to the door," Tatiana suggested. We watched from the car as she climbed the concrete stairs to bang on the door. It was the end of October and winter was near. It was a miserable, wet day as Tatiana pulled her coat tighter, looking up, and banged again. Grabbing her phone from her pocket, she made a call as she came back to the car for warmth.

"Alright, they are coming. Follow me." At the door I could hear heavy metal keys rattling against the door. It opened wide and a woman wearing her white coat with hair pulled back quickly walked away. So much for a friendly hello.

We entered to find the most beautiful grand staircase. We didn't go up, but instead were brought around and under to a colorful playroom with toys galore. Indigo blue wallpaper covered with bright, floor to ceiling gold stars inviting us in to play. Gymnastic shapes to tumble on, puppets to pretend with, rocking chairs, and books. Yes, this place was very different. There was even a ball pit in the corner. I hoped the people cared about the children as much as the building.

With that thought, in came Bogdana. She was beautiful, only nineteen months old. She was tall and looked so healthy. They handed her to me, and I could immediately feel the weight difference between her and Nikita. She had round, chubby cheeks to go with her big brown eyes. Healthy hair that had already been cut into a little bob, or more like a bowl cut, trimmed and short. Dressed to a tee in a red dress, white tights, and dress shoes.

Bogdana wasn't scared. She didn't have much of a reaction at all, really. I sat back down with her on my lap, facing me. She was smiling and happy. Much more mobile and healthier than Nikita, but still so close in age.

"Do you think she looks healthy?" Michael asked.

"She's definitely well fed!" I laughed. "I don't see

anything that jumps out at me. She is attentive and happy. Her upper lip shows no signs of fetal alcohol syndrome."

"What about the chronic health problems?" Michael worried.

"She has a clear medical history besides that, that's the only thing that scares me too, but everything I've read says it's not always passed down. Bogdana's medical says she is negative of everything."

I played and loved on her, while Michael watched and rolled a ball back and forth. Bogdana was special, but something was different for me, and Michael could tell.

"What are you thinking?" He asked me the familiar question, getting right to the point.

"I don't know, Michael. They are only five months apart," I said.

"Is that all that's bothering you? We can't leave her here," He said.

"That's not fair to say." I objected

"Well, that's what we are doing if we don't take her." Michael said. I looked at her sweet face and felt terrible. I couldn't completely explain my feelings or understand them myself, but there was caution in my mind. I had no immediate connection like I had with Nikita, or even a desire to bond like I had with Yegor and Krishina. I couldn't put my finger on it, but there was something missing.

"GOD'S GIFT." Tatiana shared the meaning of Bogdana's name on the way home. I pondered that, thinking about what life would be like with two toddlers. I would be the one returning to work. The kids are only five months apart, that would be a huge undertaking for Michael.

Is she our gift? The question floated in my mind. Bogdana was wonderful, but there was something missing. I didn't have that connection like I did with Nikita, but there were still feelings for her. Maybe feelings somewhere between motherly instinct and obligation.

All of a sudden, Tatiana's dad pulled off the road and got out of the car. We were in the middle of nowhere. So where was he going?

"Mushrooms." Tatiana looked back and smiled. She must have been able to tell we were confused. "He is buying mushrooms from that lady there."

"Lucky for your dad."

"Oh, yes, he loves mushrooms!" We all laughed as he walked back with a huge smile, put the treasure in the trunk, and with a little chuckle under his breath, got in and off we went again.

Back on the Kaliningrad streets, we pulled up to the hotel. Tatiana bid her father farewell and got out with us.

"You talk about children. I come to your hotel room tomorrow evening seven o'clock to hear decision. Da." Tatiana was all business.

"Da, see you tomorrow. Thank you," I said. She turned, walking down the sidewalk into the darkness.

"I wonder where she goes." Michael asked.

"I know, it's like she just shows up and then leaves into the night. Our own personal superhero," I laughed. Tatiana did have a mysterious way about her. We knew she had a car, but after the first trip we seldom saw her driving. People walk a lot in Russia.

CHAPTER SEVENTEEN

I thought my life had ended losing Yegor and Krishina, but as God's plan unfolded in my lap, I stood in awe of Him. The past three days had been exhausting, but the Russian people had been so kind and caring to us. I was overwhelmed by the unique way God turned this devastating situation into something good. And now, we had to make a life altering decision for us and these children.

We had been up all night arguing. I had so many mixed feelings, but Michael was certain we couldn't leave Bogdana behind. I loved how much he had done a complete 180 from where we began. Just over a year ago, he was dead-set against adoption; now he wanted to take them all home. We both finally fell asleep by five in the morning. There was no hurry getting up early, and the sun wouldn't rise until at least 10:00a.m. We just didn't want to miss lunch with our American friends.

TWO OTHER COUPLES, also adopting, joined us for lunch. Both couples had amazing stories about their children and reasons for coming. One couple, Jenny and Scott, beamed like brand new parents talking about what their new family would look like.

"The girls are five and seven," Jenny said.

"Are they full siblings?" I asked.

"Yes, they are so sweet. Here they are during our last visit." Jenny proudly shared pictures of her girls. We learned that the girls would soon have two big brothers who were also adopted from Russia years ago.

"So you met a boy and a girl?" Scott asked.

"We did, the boy on Friday and the girl yesterday," I shared.

"Siblings?"

"No, only five months apart."

"Well, they're siblings now, they just don't know it yet!" Scott laughed. He meant well by his comment, but Michael and I exchanged a look. I was still so unsure of what to do. I laughed with everyone to keep conversation light, but my stomach turned at the decision that would need to be made.

Lindsey and Allan were there adopting the daughter they had always wanted. This wasn't their first time either. They also had a son adopted from Russia. We chatted about our kids. They were all wondering about our last court date, and we talked about how hard it was to lose Yegor and Krishina.

I loved this time, sharing stories with others who understood adoption, understood the deep desire of having a family, the sadness of every situation, and the trials and risks of it all. Adoption is hard, harder than I ever imagined, but these couples understood.

We chatted over lunch about medical concerns and language barriers. Jenny and Scott were going to live here during the waiting period after court. They had an apartment picked out nearby and were doing their best to immerse themselves in the language.

"We will be here the whole month of December and will be able to pick up the girls during the waiting period because we aren't leaving the country," Scott said. "If any of you are here in December, you can come visit."

It was amazing, really, how committed we all had to be to bringing these children into our families. Trying our best to acclimate our lives for them. Adoption is not about the parents, it's about the kids—what they need to feel comfortable, safe, and loved.

We parted ways with Scott and his wife, but Allan and Lindsey were up for sightseeing. It was a beautiful day, and we needed to clear our minds of the decision ahead. Bill had heard of a WWII submarine museum that we could tour, and Michael was willing to walk just to see it.

Kaliningrad in October could not have been prettier. The sun was warm and the sky was a perfect blue. We strolled the streets toward the port, taking pictures along the way. How good it felt to have some normalcy to this trip. Past the busy city streets was a park; the lawn was manicured, and the sidewalks led to an adorable arched bridge. I talked with Lindsey about the kids, and I opened up about not being sure. Our conversation flowed like old friends.

"Have you guys been to the open air market yet?" Lindsey asked.

I looked at her with questioning eyes. "Um, no."

"Oh, you have to go. It's behind the Cathedral on Victory square," Lindsey said, and I made a mental note to make time for that. Lindsey went on sharing about her son and how good he was at soccer. We heard our husbands talking about the history of WWII. It was all so normal, and it was nice.

When we finally returned to the hotel, I convinced Michael to take one last outing to the market. I wasn't ready to tackle the decision that still loomed ahead. Past the cathedral in Victory Square, we strolled the unfamiliar path, hoping to find the market Lindsey had told me about. Just as I was beginning to get scared, the skyline cleared and a field of lean-to shacks with tin roofs appeared. The place was sketchy, at best, and I was glad Michael was carrying all the money.

We entered the rows and rows of booths, much like an American flea market, but dirtier and smellier. The sight of fish on ice, with the gut buckets nearby, suggested how fresh it really was. If the smell didn't turn your stomach, it would make a nice meal. At the sight of full pigs, head and all, hanging on butcher racks, I decided I was done. I needed out before I threw up.

We quickly headed the opposite direction from the sights and smells, finding handmade quilts, jewelry, and trinkets. I found the most adorable handmade aprons that I snatched up for no more than a dollar a piece. Booth after booth of authentic Russian souvenirs. Women, young and old, were running many of the booths, while children would run past chasing each other. Sometimes there would be a child selling things from an upturned bucket, begging for our attention.

"Ya ne govoru, Angliskiy Plesasta," I would say, so thankful Scott and Jenny had taught us how to say, "I don't speak Russian, English please."

We walked on, collecting hats, jewelry, and my favorite, matryoshka dolls, and some DVDs with Russian cartoons. After we had more than we could carry, we decided it was time to head back.

Walking back to our hotel, we spotted a Subway restaurant. We were so hungry, and the thought of having another American option excited our taste buds. As the door swung open, the smell of warm bread and a tinge of fish welcomed us. With all the treasures I found, I forgot how hungry I was. I overlooked the fish smell and was excited to get my usual chicken and bacon.

We both unwrapped our subs that we had to point out every item we wanted on them. With the first bite, I knew something was wrong. I looked at Michael, he was wearing the same disgusted face.

"Does your sandwich taste spoiled?" I asked.

"It's not a spoiled taste." He smelled it as he gagged to himself. I bravely took another bite, "Oh no, I can't. It's anchovies." I lifted the sandwich and smelled the mayo. "I think it's the mayo. It must have anchovies in it."

"I can't finish this. I'd rather go back to McDonalds," Michael said, and I agreed.

THE EVENTS of the day wore us out and we found ourselves resting in our hotel room and talking about what would come. The decision I had avoided all day. We still didn't agree, but Tatiana would need an answer.

"Michael, she is healthy. Someone will take her. I'm just not sure that it should be us. We don't even know what our little boy will need medically."

"So, you are 100% about him."

"Yes, I am," I said with authority.

"I agree, but I can't imagine leaving her after we have met her."

"I know, I would love to take her too, but they are only five months apart. You understand that would be like having twins, right? Are you ready for that? Because I'll be going back to work after maternity leave, and you will be home taking care of them!" and with that, there was a knock at the door. Michael answered the door to let Tatiana in.

"Hello, Morgan family. Have you decided what children you would like?" Tatiana asked with a smile on her face, like today was no different, and a life-changing decision for everyone involved didn't have to be made.

"We are a little undecided," I said. "We definitely want the little boy, but haven't decided yet about the girl."

"I see, we need a decision as soon as possible so I can get paperwork started."

"We understand."

"Would you like to visit her again tomorrow?" Tatiana offered. We looked at each other, not knowing that was an option. I shrugged my shoulder, looking at Michael with raised brows.

"Maybe that would help," Michael said.

"Very well, I'll make those arrangements, and then you decide tomorrow. I go next door to talk with other couple if you need me."

"Will we be able to see Nikita before we leave?" I quickly asked.

"No, unfortunately there is no time left." Tatiana looked between us. Michael nodded his head to go forward with the plan.

The door closed behind her at the same time my eyes closed in true grief. This was torture. How could we make a decision and know that we were doing the right thing for all of us?

"Well, okay." Michael was satisfied with the plan.

My eyes were still closed, begging God for an answer. I was sitting next to an invisible fireplace, heat washed over my body. Wind sucked the sheer curtains out the open window. I felt at peace.

"My plans are laid out, daughter. She is not yours. Go visit your boy one last time."

"So, we go visit her tomor--"

"She isn't ours, Michael. She isn't meant for us. And the thought of leaving here without seeing Nikita again; I can't do it." I was certain this was the right answer.

"Are you sure?" Michael questioned.

"Yes, I am. I have peace that she's healthy, and she will get picked."

"Okay, you sound pretty sure. If that's what you really want, I'll support you." Michael held out his hands, "You're sure?" Looking straight in his eyes, I nodded my head.

Lord, you know our story from beginning to end. Confirm in our hearts what is next, show us what to do. Again I felt a peace that comes only from God, *My plans are laid out daughter. She is not yours.*

"She isn't ours, Michael. Go tell Tatiana before we change our mind." I motioned him out the door.

Michael knocked on the neighbor's door. Lindsey and Allan were also on their second trip, and they were heading to court for adoption instead of stopping an adoption.

"Michael, you need me?" Tatiana said.

"Yes, could you stop by our room after you are finished?"

"Da, of course," she nodded and closed the door.

Moments later, Tatiana returned looking a bit sad, or maybe tired; either one was not like herself.

"How can I do for you?" Tatiana looked concerned. It was late on a Sunday evening. I knew she was missing her family time to coordinate everyone else's.

"Are you okay?" I asked out of concern. I was sure the stress of the job had to affect her eventually.

"Oh, yes, I will be fine. What can I do here? You make decision?" Tatiana asked.

"We decided to only adopt the little boy and would like to go see him tomorrow," Michael said.

"For sure, that is wonderful news. Congratulations!" Tatiana smiled and hugged me. "I will have driver here at 9:00a.m. to take you to Gusev." The weight of the decision was lifted.

"That is such good news after having to tell Allan and Lindsey they adoption was stopped," Tatiana added.

"Their adoption fell through?" I repeated, glancing at Michael.

"Da, it is sad. I had just told them the news before you knocked. It is not normal, but happy for you both. He is such beautiful baby! I'll see you tomorrow." Tatiana turned and was out the door.

I realized God had moved at that very moment. The moment Allan and Lindsey were getting this terrible news, I was reassured that Bogdana was not ours, that she belonged to someone else, possibly to them. The Holy Spirit guided us at that very moment.

*"Jesus replied, 'You do not realize now what I am doing,
but later you will understand.'"*
John 13:7

WE HEADED down to breakfast the next morning ready for the day, but we knew Allan and Lindsey would not be.

"Are you guys okay?" I asked as we sat down with them.

"Our adoption fell through," Allan said.

"I'm so sorry. We heard that. Was it family like our case?" I asked.

"We are not sure at this point. Tatiana said she would know more today, but that we could see other girls if they had any available," Allan went on. I could see the pain on Lindsey's face, she was trying not to cry. I knew that pain far too well.

"I don't know if this is a possibility, but we decided to only adopt our boy. Maybe you can visit Bogdana, the little girl, today?"

Hope shined in Lindsey's eyes, "Really?"

"Yes, really. We decided at the same time you got your news. That's why Michael knocked on your door," I said.

"Do you have any pictures of her?" Lindsey asked.

"I do." We both leaned in close while I pulled up pictures and video from my camera and shared what medical information we knew. Neither of us knew if Bogdana was even a possibility for them, but I knew last night was not a coincidence.

"Be joyful in hope, patient in affliction, faithful in prayer."
Romans 12:12

IT WAS afternoon before we reached Gusev. Our last meal was breakfast, but I was getting used to only eating sporadically and carrying extra snacks. Getting back to our son was top on my survival list, even above eating. Seeing him this last time before we left would give me strength to leave without him.

When they carried him in, he was just as perfect as I remembered. His thin hair brushed smooth, wearing a baby blue fleece sleeper. Not as scared as our first meeting, but still cautious. I wasted no time getting the toys out. We played on the floor with stacking balls and things that rattled. He loved feeling the softness of the blanket we had brought, using it to cover his head to play peek-a-boo, and wouldn't let it go.

There were no worries about him getting into anything. He wasn't crawling and liked to lay on his belly. Definitely right handed, he would rest on his left elbow while moving toys with his right. If he was sitting up, he stayed clung to my fingers for support, but Michael was taking on a whole new role as playmate. I loved watching them on the floor, Michael playing airplane, holding him high in the air, seeing the first genuine smiles from our now favorite boy in the whole world. I so admired my husband, and fatherhood looked amazing on him.

Before long, Nikita began to tire. His little ten-month-old body needed a nap as he self-soothed, sucking his thumb and rocking back and forth. I couldn't bear to let him rock himself when my heart ached to do nothing more than that.

I scooped him up and cradled him in my arms as he snuggled up against my soft fleece vest. He sucked his thumb as we rocked, and I felt his body relax and quietly fall asleep in my arms. Here I was in Gusev, Russia, holding my baby boy. Gratitude washed over me.

"Are you happy?" Michael asked. He had been watching this moment unfold while I was in my own world. Finally, the moment I had been waiting for, the moment that I truly felt like a mom. I looked up at him with tears I couldn't wipe because my hands were so full.

"Yes. Very."

Driving back to Kaliningrad was heavy. I had just left my son behind, and I was worried about Bogdana. *Had we made the right decision? Did Allan and Lindsey get to meet her today?* Tatiana drove quickly, and she began to discuss what would come next.

"I will have everything ready. It looks like court will be

on December 20 or 21. You will need to come early to spend at least five days with baby for bonding time."

"And is there a possibility for this to fall through like our first?" I asked.

"There is always chance, but Inga said there is no family close. Only uncle in Moscow, but he is not married and does not want kids. So much less chance, do not worry."

"What will you name him?" Tatiana asked.

I had been waiting for this question. Neither of us wanted to use the name Maverick. That name had already been taken, and he didn't look like a Maverick either. My mom had suggested a name months ago that we both liked. It didn't fit before now, but now it was perfect.

I smiled, "His name is Rush."

"But now, this is what the Lord says...Fear not, for I have redeemed you; I have summoned you by name; you are mine."
Isaiah 43:1

"WE ARE ADOPTING BOGDANA!" Lindsey looked full of hope as we all sat down for dinner.

"So you did get to visit her today! I am so relieved, I have been worrying about you all day."

"We did, we asked Tatiana about her first thing this morning. She is perfect!" Lindsey was so excited.

"That's great news! The crazy part is, I think she looks like you guys!" I smiled. "And we should be traveling back at the same time." I was so excited for them, and I was so glad I listened to the caution of the Holy Spirit. In the moment, I felt the responsibility of the situation, Michael's persistence, and my own desires to bring them both home with me. I could have ignored that small voice, but it would not have been God's plan. I would not have been able to see the joy on Lindsey's face tonight, felt the peace of making the right choice, or even held Rush one last time before leaving. *Thank you, Jesus, for loving me.*

"Do not be anxious about anything, but in every situation, by prayer and petition, with thanksgiving, present your request to God. And the peace of God, which transcends all understanding, will guard your hearts and your minds in Christ Jesus."
Philippians 4:6-7

CHAPTER EIGHTEEN

The decision was made. We would have a son by next year, possibly Christmas, but of course, we would have to make two more trips. By the time we arrived home, a court date was set. Tatiana had hoped we could get him home before January, but because Russians celebrate New Year's, then Christmas on January seventh, everyone takes two weeks off in January. If we had to wait, it would be mid-January before bringing him home. For now the hardest part was upon us, the wait.

Sadly, I couldn't shake the feeling that this was too good to be true. Was I even deserving of this fairy-tale ending? I had questioned God way too much. I lost faith in his power. I had truly underestimated Him, and yet I had never needed Him so much in my whole life.

From my window seat on the plane, I lowered my head into my hands.

Father, forgive me. Forgive me for not trusting. My whole

life I've kept you in a neat little box, but you are so much greater than that. I'm not worthy of this ending. The silence in my mind filled, *Daughter, I have always loved you more than you loved me. You will never surpass the love I have for you! Accept this gift freely.* I looked up with tears in my eyes.

"Are you okay?" Michael asked.

I sniffed, nodding my head. "It's all just sinking in right now. I'm just thinking about how mad I was at God. It's embarrassing, and how my whole life I've loved Him, but I never knew Him. You know? I've never needed Him to fix a situation or solve a problem before now."

"Some things are out of our control." Michael reached for my hand to hold.

"I know, but I've always thought that if I made the right choices, it didn't have to be out of my control! Like God has rewarded me because I made good choices, but it's not like that! God's not like that. This was his plan from the beginning."

"Well, God is not Santa Claus, Samantha!" Michael laughed.

"I know," I said while hitting his shoulder. "I never realized God would love me, or love anybody, with nothing in return."

"What was the point of Jesus dying on the cross then? His resurrection would mean nothing if you had a to-do list for Him to love you," Michael said.

"I guess I never fully grasped that idea. That He loves me even when I mess up. He loves me through the hard stuff. I guess I always thought, because I had a list of good deeds, I would always be on his nice list. Okay, yeah, it kind of sounds like Santa Claus!" I chuckled at the thought.

"Um, yeah. You think?" Michael smiled.

I had a new grace-filled relationship with God, a newfound trust. I realized I served a God who loves me unconditionally, His forgiveness overflows. I didn't need to always be perfect to gain His love, but my desire to do good isn't based on reward. I want to do good and make Him proud, not because I might get something, but because I love Him, and I am grateful for His unconditional forgiveness and grace. I want to be worthy of Jesus's sacrifice for me, even though I don't deserve it and never will.

"Praise be to the God and Father of our Lord Jesus Christ! In his great mercy he has given us new birth into a living hope through the resurrection of Jesus Christ from the dead,"
1 Peter 1:3

THE FLIGHT HOME gave us plenty of time to reminisce and dream of our future with Rush. There were opportunities to connect with our family page, but I never did. At least for the next fourteen hours, we would keep him to ourselves. I had forgotten my camera cord at home and couldn't post pictures even if I wanted to. The family page hadn't even been updated about Rush and just how miraculous this trip had been. I knew everyone would be wondering, but I would save that post until we got home. I smiled, thinking that this was our moment, and he was our gift from God.

Arriving home in the middle of the night, I couldn't wait any longer. Michael fell asleep immediately, but I could sleep all day tomorrow, so I wrote.

OCTOBER 27

HOME SWEET HOME! What a crazy week in Russia. We feel good about what God has for our lives. We will not be posting pictures on Facebook for the world to see this time. If I feel like it later, I might post one here to the family page. Through our trials, we have witnessed God at work placing children without homes into families who will love them. Yegor and Krishina will be living with their aunt. We met two children this trip and decided to only adopt one. However, the other family that was there saw her picture, and now they will be adopting the girl we did not choose, as well as waiting to adopt the first child they were there for. We will be adopting a 10 month old boy, he will be one in two months. Four kids finding homes. God knew what He was doing. Thank you all for the prayers...they got us through this tough time.

I FOUND THE CAMERA CORD, smiling as I scrolled through my pictures. Rush was perfect for us, and God knew he belonged here in my arms.

OCTOBER 27

This is all you get.

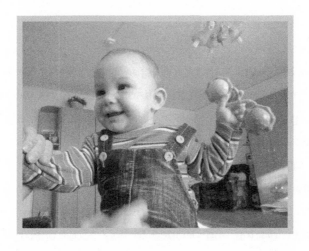

THE NEXT FEW months were nerve racking. I knew there was a possibility of losing Rush, but I tried to busy myself with school and planning for yet another substitute teacher. My resilient fifth graders were handling my absence in stride. They were excited for me. My identity for so long had only been the teacher, but I was finally going to experience the other side. I had waited so long to be a mom, it didn't seem real. Travel arrangements were made and the countdown had begun. I updated the family with the official plans.

NOVEMBER 21,

Court date is set. If all goes well, it will be final on December 29th! This trip, we should be home December 21st. We have to make one more trip the second week in January to pick Rush up. And I had to post just one more picture.

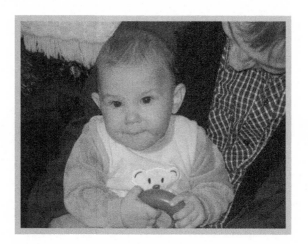

THE WEEK before court would be our time to bond with Rush. We would arrive the day after his first birthday, and I could hardly wait to spend that week with him. His first birthday party was in the works as I picked out the perfect packable presents and everything but the cake.

I tried my best to keep the voices in my head at bay, but whispers still reminded me that his biological family would be notified, and it could, it might, all fall apart. I had to remind myself that those voices were not from God. The devil had tried his best to destroy my peace, but I found myself falling deeper in love with Jesus.

"Jesus said to him, 'Away from me, Satan! For it is written: 'Worship the Lord your God, and serve him only.' Then the devil left him, and angels came and attended him."
Matthew 4:10-11

CHAPTER NINETEEN

"Um, I thought you were packing?" Michael laughed.

I sat in the middle of our bedroom floor with every article of clothing laid out in front, beside, and behind me. Everywhere, actually, but in the suitcase. Frantically packing, I was making sure all the socks and underwear were accounted for.

"I don't want to forget anything. I started to pack and then forgot what I had packed. Just keep walking; this makes complete sense to me!" I smirked and waved my hand to excuse him.

We had gotten an email that everything was fine. All the family had been contacted and no one had come forward to stop the adoption. I was in a much better place this trip than last. I couldn't wait to get back to my baby. I finally zipped the suitcase and placed it by the door to wait until morning.

DECEMBER 12,

Not sure if we are ready for tomorrow, but we are prepared! We should get to St. Petersburg Tuesday around 4:00p.m. Pray we don't miss any planes this time. Love you all.

ANOTHER QUICK TRIP TO ST. Petersburg brought nasty weather. About what I expected December in Russia to be like: cold. We were here for medical exams, again. But, thank the Lord, this time we only signed a few papers and were able to use our last medical evaluations. I hadn't messed anything up this time. Today was Rush's first birthday. It killed me not being with him, but at least we were in the same country. We would get to see him and celebrate tomorrow.

DECEMBER 15

We made it with no problems. We were met in St. Pete yesterday with snow and soggy weather. Medicals are done...again (very easy the second time). Just waiting to fly to Kaliningrad. The sun did not come up here until after 11am! How depressing, I couldn't live here! Ready to have a birthday party tomorrow!

TRAVELING HAD BECOME like second nature to us. We hurried everywhere just to sit and wait, but this trip I was worried about Michael.

"Are you okay? You don't look so good. Are you car sick?" I asked. He was turning pale as we began to land in Kaliningrad.

"I don't know what's wrong, but no, I don't feel good at all." Michael closed his eyes and leaned his head back. I felt so bad for him, but there was nothing I could do. Jet lag was real and, maybe after traveling around the world three times it was starting to show.

Back in Kaliningrad, we settled into our familiar hotel room. Michael still felt sick, but I had a birthday party to throw. We walked down the cold street to our favorite bistro just a few blocks from our hotel. I needed a birthday cake and remembered them having a small bakery. If comfort had a smell, this would be it. Warm vanilla, melted sugars, and bread captured my senses.

Perfectly baked bear claws, cinnamon rolls, and sweets I had never seen waited proudly. I scanned each pastry behind the glass case until my eyes rested on a small chocolate mouse. Its body was just bigger than a cake pop, with a Hersey kiss for the head, crowned with little chocolate chip ears and a snowflake on its back. That was it! That little mouse would be a perfect smash cake for a one-year-old.

I smiled at the girl and pointed to the little mouse. As

she pointed to it I said, "Yes, da." She pulled it out and placed it in a small white travel box. Michael paid and we headed back to the hotel. The street lights were returning for the evening as we jumped over puddles.

"So you have a birthday cake, what else do you need?" Michael knew I had a plan.

"Actually, nothing! I have a party hat, a number one candle, and his presents. I even brought the gift bags in my suitcase!" I smiled. "This weather's got nothing on me!"

I was so thankful and had such an appreciation for that word. I was so full of thanks. I gazed at each person in our friends and family page, thankful for each of them, among so many other things.

DECEMBER 15

As I look through the members in this group, I can't help but feel blessed you are all in our lives!

"Perfume and incense bring joy to the heart,
and the pleasantness of one's friend
springs from his earnest counsel."
Proverbs 27:9

THERE WAS no way this hotel would have us back. As we waited for Elina to return, the pit in my stomach was growing. I was still embarrassed by our messy room and knew they would say no.

Elina jumped back in the car. "They say they have no room," she said. I gave Michael a sideways glance. He knew what I was thinking.

"There one more hotel around corner." Peeling around the square, Elina barely looked as she pulled out. We were at the next hotel in a flash, and she was out the door.

"She doesn't look happy," Michael noticed as she headed back to the car. Elina sat sideways in the front seat to see us in the back.

"They say they do not have room again, but they do," Elina said.

"Well, that's disappointing," I said.

"They are afraid hotel will not be good enough for Americans. Do you want to stay here or stay in Kaliningrad?"

"I don't want to drive from Kaliningrad every day! I don't care what the hotel is like." I spoke for both of us.

Elina nodded her head, "Let me ask again," and off she went.

"I'd be even sicker if we drove every day," Michael added. Within a few minutes she was back. Elina must have amazing negotiating skills, because we were unloading our suitcases and heading in.

"They found best room for you. We drop off your things, and I will take you to orphanage."

Up two flights of stairs, we opened the front door, dropped everything into the dark hotel room, and turned back around to get to my baby boy.

It was only four o'clock in the afternoon, but the sun was already setting. A mere six hours of sunlight was all this little town was getting. It didn't matter one bit to me, I wasn't here for the weather. I slid my backpack off and laid the green and blue birthday bags at my feet as we sat on the couch to wait.

Six agonizing weeks to get back to my baby; I couldn't take much more. My knee bounced, but Michael laid his hand there, calming my nerves. Finally, the nurse walked in with my little guy. A year old yesterday, he had changed so much! His little cheeks were plump, and his hair was growing thicker. The workers had him dressed in jeans and a striped orange and brown shirt that made him look so big. His little toes, covered by blue socks, showed through the blue leather sandals.

I stood, reaching for him immediately. Wrapping him in my arms, I breathed him in.

"Happy Birthday, big guy!" I smiled, assuring his worried look that everything would be okay. He wasn't sure, and definitely didn't remember us, but who could blame him. The weight of him in my arms filled in years of waiting, praying, and tears. As if God was telling me, *See, this is what you have been waiting for. No other child would do; out of the whole world, I handpicked him for you and you for him.*

He was so unsure of what was happening, and that's

when the tears came. I knew this was a possibility, so I just hugged and loved on him, doing my best to calm his nerves.

"I wonder how often he even leaves the baby room." I looked Michael's way with the open ended question. "This could all be new, not just us."

"Maybe," was all Michael offered.

I held him tight, rocking him until the tears stopped and his breathing returned to normal. Wanting a better look at my son, I sat down crisscross applesauce on the floor with Rush perched on my right leg, protected tightly under my arm. Once he was attached, he wasn't letting go, so we rocked and talked. I kissed his soft head, and with him close to my heart, we started breathing at the same time. Rush took a little peek up at me with his big brown eyes, wanting to trust me.

"Mama's here, baby," I said. His little chubby cheeks were full, and I thought I saw his two bottom teeth. He had gotten so big in the past two months. With him much more comfortable in his surroundings, I stood him directly in front of me. He was standing much better with support, even though he wasn't using his legs as much as we would like.

After Rush was ready to explore, Michael set up the camera to capture his birthday party. That was top on my priority list, and I loved that we wouldn't miss his first.

Inga's office was more private with only one working nurse. I pulled out the party supplies, placed the hat on Rush's head, and took out the little cake. I didn't think to bring a plate, so I placed it in the palm of my hand. Sadly, I had forgotten the little candle, so I readied my little family for pictures without it.

He had no idea what was going on. The nurse smiled, probably laughing at our over-the-top American traditions. Looking up from the floor, I spoke to the woman behind the desk.

"Can he taste this?" She didn't understand me, so I pointed to the cake and then to Rush, hoping she would understand.

"Nyet, Nyet. Too young," she replied with a disapproving head shake, obviously not pleased with my parenting skills.

"Well, there goes your birthday smash cake," I whispered in Rush's ear, not that he cared in the slightest. I held the little cake in the palm of my left hand while Michael held Rush. We sang happy birthday, took a few pictures, and then I placed the mouse cake back in the box. If he couldn't eat it, I would enjoy it later.

Rush was so cute with his little party hat. He was still not sitting up well enough on his own, so I plopped him in my lap to open his presents. A bright green bag with sparkly polka dots and blue tissue paper was exactly what he didn't know he wanted for his birthday.

The glitter dots on the gift bag had his attention. They were rough to the touch and just the right amount of sparkle. We finally coaxed him to pull out the blue sensory elephant and little toddler toy balls, or I should say, I finally dumped them out. He was no more excited than before, so we let him keep playing with the bag.

He was so stoic, and one of the only smiles I was able to get was with that silly bag. He was trying to crawl, but still not walking or standing. As Rush lay on the floor, his legs twisted, Michael pulled his jeans to untangle his limp legs. This was concerning, but we believed that encouragement and room to move would grow his confidence. With love and attention and possibly physical therapy, he would take right off.

Moving forward we start bonding and learning together as a family. We had a whole week ahead of us to do nothing but concentrate on our boy. Even if Rush was scared right now, I knew that he would start recognizing us soon, just as Yegor and Krishina did.

"We have this hope as an anchor for the soul, firm and secure. It enters the inner sanctuary behind the curtain,"
Hebrews 6:19

THE WALK back to the hotel was nice. It was dark, but the moon was full and the street lamps lit the way. We walked the familiar path, turning at the same grocery store. It was cold, but we were prepared. Layers of clothing under our heavy winter coats kept us warm. We knew Russia would be cold in December.

I was so exhausted. All I wanted to do was sleep, and Michael didn't look well. We reached the age old rock building and ascended the stairs to the top floor.

Michael turned the heavy gold key, and we both scampered around in the pitch dark searching for a light switch. Only a few feet into the room and I hit a wall. For some reason, it felt like a hallway instead of a bedroom.

"Found it!" I yelled, and as the lights came on, we could only stare at each other. We were in a hallway, or maybe an entryway.

"This looks interesting," I smiled at yet another adventure unfolding. The orange shag carpet went two ways, so we split up to explore. Finding light switches as I went to the left of the front door, the carpet led to a living room with a couch and a chair that could have been in my grandmother's home, a box TV, and another doorway.

Through the doorway, Michael was already laying on the large bed crowned with two side tables, each with a lamp.

"What's through there?" I asked, pointing to the doorway across the room.

"The bathroom," Michael offered. I continued on around through the bathroom until I found myself back in the entryway. This was no ordinary hotel room. They had treated us with the nicest apartment they had. Although dated, it was roomy and had a great view of the square. Even though it would be dark and dreary most of the time, it was still nice of them. The Wi-Fi signal was weak, but I was still able to update the family.

DECEMBER 16

They wouldn't let him eat his birthday cake, and the nurse thought I was crazy for still wanting to take a picture with it! If you can't tell, it's a little mouse with a snowflake on top. (I forgot the #1 candle I bought for it).

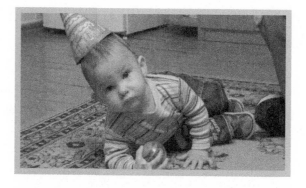

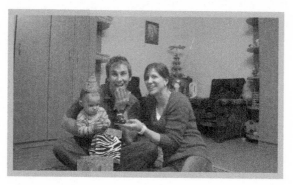

"I'M SO READY TO SLEEP," I said as I shut the computer and rolled over to find Michael snoring with a pillow over his head. "Well, I guess you are too," I chuckled to myself.

I couldn't have slept more than a few hours, tossing and turning all night. This was a nice apartment, but the mattress was terrible. By the time Michael woke, I had posted to the group again.

DECEMBER 16,

He has gotten so big in 6 weeks. 2 bottom teeth, 2 top will probably come in a month or less. Not walking yet, but he is much more mobile than before. Can stand (kind of) by himself. I can tell he wants to, he will probably just start running soon. Tatianna said no problems and hopes Monday (court) comes and goes uneventfully and quickly.

CHAPTER TWENTY

After Rush's birthday party, I hoped he would recognize us. *Lord, let Rush remember us. Let me become his safe place.*

He looked happier as they placed him in my arms. No tears, yet. Today was already better than yesterday. I didn't want to do anything the workers would think was unusual, so we played with our toys on the floor. I never realized the strange things we do with babies until we were being observed. I wanted to make him laugh, making silly faces and noises, but knew I would look like a clown. I had no idea what the workers would think of us, and I didn't want to do anything they thought was wrong. Before we knew it, our time was up, and we could come back in the afternoon.

We enjoyed the space of our little apartment, and I kept the family up to date from Facebook.

December 17

We are staying in Gusev (the same town as the orphanage, and the same orphanage as last time). We can walk there 2 times a day. We saw him this morning, and he was happier to see us. I hope he will start to recognize us soon. He cried for the majority of the time yesterday.

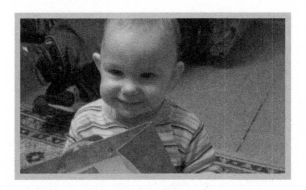

THE WEEK CONTINUED to get better, and the workers quickly trusted us, giving us more privacy in Inga's office. I did the normal things that seemed odd with someone watching. I took Rush's shoes and socks off to count his little toes and tickle his little feet. We played peek-a-boo, and I blew on his big cheeks and belly, making noises. That finally gave me the belly laugh of my dreams. He was so adorable, the cutest baby to ever live.

We moved those little legs of his and made him stand. This time was so important for him to gain strength and start pulling up and standing on his own. He needed this one-on-one attention, and I could tell he loved it.

Like a game, he would wiggle his way between the heavy wooden chairs. I would laugh and say, "Where is Rush Nikita?" Finally comfortable to play and laugh, I would slide him out on the wooden floor just for him to do it all over again.

Michael watched but kept his distance. His eyes sunken and dark, still clearly sick.

"I'm sorry you can't enjoy this," I said.

"I enjoy watching you," he said sweetly. We knew our time was coming to a close when a busty nurse with out-of-the-box bright red hair walked in. Rush saw her and his eyes lit up.

"Moi mal'chik Nikita, prishol," she said, smiling big with no front teeth. I had always worried if he could bond to us with never bonding before, but he clearly loved this worker and she loved him. She scooped him up with a big hug and with Rush's hand, she waved goodbye to us. That sweet woman was who I had been praying for to look after and love my son until I returned.

"This is the confidence we have in approaching God: that if we ask anything according to his will, he hears us. And if we know that he hears us--whatever we ask--we know that we have what we asked of him."
1 John 5:14-15

DECEMBER 17

Today was different, he was very happy today. Pray for Michael, he is sick. Sleeps every extra bit he can. I'm sitting in the café by myself right now so he can sleep. Hopefully I will post again soon! And, yep, 10 fingers and toes! We checked...also an outie belly button.

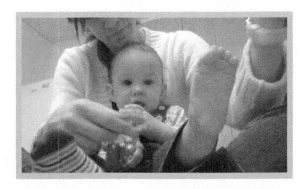

I UPDATED the family before taking a nap. Nights had been restless. I tried to sleep, but I felt like the princess and the pea. Something was wrong with the mattress.

"Are you sleeping well at night?' I asked Michael.

"No, the bed is hard as a rock," Michael agreed. "I sleep better on the couch," he said. I decided to investigate, lifting the layers of sheets to find a block of wood covered in orange fabric. Nestled in the wooden bed was a two inch pallet tufted with buttons like the back of a couch. That was our mattress.

"Okay, no wonder this bed is so hard, it's not really a mattress," I said in shock.

THE MOMENT THEY WALKED IN, I knew something was different. Between our two trips and time at this orphanage, we had become quite comfortable with the coming and goings happening around us, but this felt different. She couldn't have been any older than me, carrying a little girl, maybe 3 years old, on her hip. As this woman spoke to the secretary, there was no emotion.

I locked eyes with Michael and nodded out the doorway for him to look. "What do you think is going on?" I asked.

"What?" Michael asked.

"That woman just walked in with a kid. It doesn't seem like a normal visit."

The secretary stood to retrieve some paperwork from the file. The woman seemed impatient, raising her hands, only to let them fall to her side with a huff. From Inga's office, we couldn't understand what was happening until the crying started. The woman put the little girl down to sign papers. The crying then escalated to screaming as the woman exited the office, nearly running away, leaving the screaming toddler. The secretary held the little girl's hand, leading her out.

"Was that a mom leaving her kid?" The situation had Michael's attention now.

"I think that's what just happened," I said. Without a translator we would never know, but body language is universal. That was sad. The confusion on that little girl's face would haunt me forever. How I just wanted to hold her. To comfort her, but it wouldn't have helped. She wanted her mother. We had struggled so hard to have a baby, and this woman left hers without looking back. *Why Lord? Why does this happen?*

*"Though my father and mother forsake me,
the Lord will receive me."
Psalm 27:10*

WE ARRIVED for our afternoon visit as usual. By now, the staff were all very comfortable with us. We played with Rush, working on his standing, crawling, and walking. Inga's office began to feel busy. There was clearly a meeting about to happen, and they didn't really want us there.

"You go. Nikita for walk, da?" Inga smiled.

"Da," I smiled. I would love to have some freedom and get some fresh air for a while. I was surprised because it was December, and I remembered how she acted in September with Yegor and Krishina outside.

"Nurse take mal'chik, change clothes." She motioned

for Rush, so I handed him over. We gathered our things and waited in the secretary's office. When he returned, he was twice the size as before, looking more like a stuffed turkey in a blue snow suit. No need for gloves, the coat was too big and his hands were nowhere in sight. A little fuzzy, knitted hat topped him off. We headed down the stairs with no instructions, no stroller, and no plan.

"What are we supposed to do?" Michael asked.

"Think we would get in trouble if we went back to our apartment?" I laughed.

"Um, yeah, I think that's a bad idea. Let's just stay around here," Michael said.

He still wasn't feeling well, and walking aimlessly has never been his favorite pastime. We followed the sidewalks around the baby home, the same paths Yegor steered his tricycle on. After a few trips, we decided to venture down the street. We walked half the block, always keeping the bright green baby home in view before turning around.

Passing us on the street was a reminder of where we were. Military soldiers marched past in perfect step. Their camo green uniforms, perfectly placed berets, and shining black AK47s, strapped and ready at their side. This was Mother Russia. We continued walking, making as little eye contact as possible.

"I'm freezing. Rush can't even move in his outfit, so I know he isn't cold, but I am," I complained. "This wind is terrible."

"I'm tired of walking, but I don't know when we can go back in," Michael said.

"Let's sit in this little house." There on the playground was a small house with bench seating inside. As soon as we were crammed inside, we found refuge from the biting wind. "I still can't believe they let us take him outside. It's so cold!" Michael said.

"I can't believe he isn't screaming or at least fussy from all the clothes they have him in." I added.

After what felt like an hour, we decided to go back. The secretary spotted us like they had all accidentally forgotten us. She let us back in, and we had Inga's office all to ourselves. One layer at a time, we peeled off Rush's outerwear. Under it all, he had on the cutest blue crocheted onesie ever. This was definitely hand made with a white ruffled collar and all.

"They even changed his underclothes to go outside!" I smiled. "I have to take more pictures." Rush was the happiest we had ever seen him. Free from his snowsuit, he started showing off his standing skills, only to slide down the wooden cabinet doors.

"Look at that ornery smile, this is the most personality I've seen," I said.

"He is going to hate these pictures someday," Michael laughed.

We played peek-a-boo from under his blanket for the rest of our time. Whatever brought the biggest smiles is what we did. He loved to walk holding my fingers, and I could tell our impromptu physical therapy was paying off.

Back in the warmth of our apartment, we thawed our toes and updated the family.

DECEMBER 18

When we went for our walk, they had to change his clothes to go outside...this was the outfit of choice! He is going to hate these pics someday. This is his 'I'm up to no good look.' We got to go for a walk for a little bit. Poor kid couldn't move with all the clothes. We get one more visit Sunday morning before we head back to get ready for court Monday.

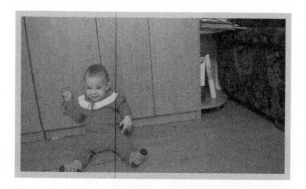

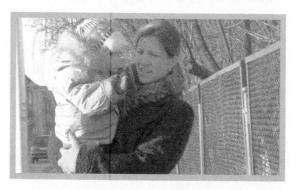

SUNDAY WAS our last visit before court. We knew to enter through the side door today because the office was closed. I knocked on the white door, hoping the nurse would invite us into the room where our son had spent his first year of life. A worker poked her head out, barely opening the door, smiled, and went back in.

"I guess they don't want us in there," I said as I joined Michael sitting on the stairs, never removing my eyes from the door; I wanted a peek, just a glimpse into my son's life. Finally, the worker emerged with Rush.

She opened the door wide enough for me to barely see inside. I looked past her, but the only thing I could see was a U shaped classroom table, similar to what I had in my classroom. The tables that a teacher could sit at and reach each child sitting around her. This table, however, had a worker at the head surrounded by babies, babies Rush's age or younger. Armed with only one spoon and one big bowl of breakfast, each little mouth was fed one right after the other, I assumed, until it was gone.

I held Rush, and we followed the nurse up the stairs. Her white uniform, from the hat to the shoes, was spotless. I wondered how she worked with babies all day and still looked so put together. She said nothing to us as she unlocked our familiar refuge. The office workers were off for the weekend, so we had the whole place to ourselves. I was free to take as many pictures as I wanted, even though

Michael still looked and felt awful. The feeling of being able to talk freely felt wonderful as well.

"Rush Nikita, Rush Nikita," I repeated his new and old name and filled the room with English. "Mamma, Mammmma." I wanted to hear those words so badly. "Dadadada. Momomom."

Before we knew it, our time was up. I held him tight as they allowed us to walk back down together, and we said our goodbyes there in the stairwell.

"Mama will be back. I love you," I whispered in his ear with a kiss. I passed him back to the nurse, quickly wiping the corners of my eyes.

DECEMBER 19

Final visit this morning. It was sad to leave him there. He watched us very closely as we headed down the stairs away from him.

CHAPTER TWENTY-ONE

Breakfast with our American friends was a welcome distraction. Today was court. Four hours to be exact, then it would be all downhill from there. Allan and Lindsey also had court for the adoption of Bogdana, who received the beautiful name of Hannah. I was so amazed how God had orchestrated each detail, and to top it all off, we would bring Rush and Hannah home together.

There was excitement in the air as we dressed for court. Instead of arriving late after devastating news and looking disheveled from a long trip, we dressed in our Sunday best. Straightening Michael's tie, I laughed. "You look good in my dad's shirt and tie."

"Well, when you spend your life savings on a family and plane tickets, you have to borrow a dress shirt and tie." He leaned down and gently kissed my forehead. After five days of jet lag and possibly food poisoning, Michael was starting to look and feel more like himself.

"I love you, Michael Morgan."

"You look pretty good yourself," he winked. I neatly tucked the maroon turtleneck into my black skirt.

"Thanks," I said. Today I would blend in with the Russian women with my tights, dark colors, and black boots.

We walked up the same courthouse steps, sat on the same uncomfortable wooden benches, but the reason we were here was totally different. The entire room had a different feel about it. This time would be a celebration.

The Judge began speaking while the secretary took notes. The caseworker and orphanage director spoke with smiles on their faces. The whole while, Michael and I looked on from our seats.

"Morgans, pozhaluysta, vstan'te," the Judge said. "Morgans, please stand." Tatiana motioned her hand for us to stand at the podium. The Judge asked several questions while Tatiana translated.

"Are you ready to parent Nikita as your son?"

We both smiled, nodded, and answered in unison, "Yes. Da."

"What activities do you do to stay active? To keep up with active boy?"

"We are both very active. I enjoy running, competitions, and dancing." I answered first, followed by Michael. "I teach Jiu Jitsu classes and boxing."

"You must eat healthy? No fast food all time?"

I laughed on the inside, thinking about all the McDonald's we had eaten while here, but back home we don't. I answered, "Yes, we try our best to cook healthy meals."

"We can tell by you size. Not all Americans are as small as you."

I blushed at the compliment, "Spasibo." Their view of American culture showed.

"Will you tell Nikita about Russia?" she asked.

"Yes, absolutely. We want him to be proud of his story, proud to be Russian. Everyone has been so kind to us, we would only have good things to tell him." I was being completely honest. I was so proud of his story, the miracle that he is, and couldn't wait to share it with him.

"Papa, what are you excited most about having boy?" The Judge directed this question at Michael, and I was anxious to hear his answer as well.

"I think I'm most excited to teach him things, like man stuff. Of course boxing and Jiu Jitsu, but also stuff like changing a tire and how to drive." As Tatiana translated, the Judge smiled big. I could tell she liked his answer, and so did I. I had never thought to ask Michael a question like that. I had been so caught up with the baby stuff; I never thought about years later or even to ask what Michael was excited about. I was still admiring my husband when Tatiana spoke to me.

"Mama, what did you notice about Nikita that only a mama would notice?" Wow, I got a tough one, and I wanted to say the right thing. I paused, thinking of our time together. He was precious for sure, but after he became comfortable with us, I could see there was more to his little personality.

"I noticed an orneriness in his eyes and an eagerness to see and learn. He also had eyes on all the ladies in the office. I'm afraid he will be quite the ladies' man." I smiled and everyone laughed.

"How did you use name Rush?" I knew the real answer was that my Mom suggested the name, and it just fit perfectly. We didn't want to use Maverick, that name had already been given to another. I tried to think of something to say that would sound better or nobler to them.

"We wanted him to keep a piece of Russia with him and thought naming him Rush would fit him and his story." I thought I had answered well, but instead they all kind of chuckled. One of the secretaries even covered her mouth with her hair to hide her laughter. I felt my neck get red under my turtleneck and thought, *I just blew it.*

Instead the Judge smiled at us and said, "Federatsiya Rossii vidit v Mikhaile i Samante Morgan pozitivnykh roditeley dya Nikita Apastlov."

Tatiana smiled and hugged us both, "She says the Federation of Russia sees Michael and Samantha Morgan as positive parents for Nikita Apastlov. Congratulations!"

I breathed a sigh of relief, "So it's done? We just have to wait to pick him up?"

"Da! We will talk more in car!" She patted both our backs. "Congratulations!"

WE SAT WAITING for Tatiana in the car, my heart full to bursting. A woman always on a mission, Tatiana slid into the driver's seat with a smile.

"Judge Petrov must like you a lot. I have never been out court so fast!" Without waiting for a response, she continued, "I have all paperwork. I will file with Secretary of Education today. There is ten day wait period before it is final, but do not worry. Family must appeal to Supreme Court in Moscow, and that would never happen. Oh, so happy for you, he is such beautiful baby! The adoption will be final December 30, but you will have to wait till after Christmas to pick him up."

"We can pick him up after Christmas or New Year's?" I was confused by Tatiana's timeline. "New Year's is January 1st, then we could fly back?"

"Oh, I am sorry. In Russia, New Year is first then Christmas is on January 7. Unfortunately, no one will be working in offices, so you will have to wait until after the Russian Christmas. Because it is Russian holiday season, it could be after Christmas in January before you can pick him up."

More waiting. The waiting is so hard, but at least there was a date to look forward to. We needed to get through the waiting period, then we could celebrate on December 30th; what a wonderful New Year it will be!

I could hardly contain my excitement as I wrote to our family and friends. I knew they wouldn't see it for hours, but I couldn't wait.

DECEMBER 20

COURT IS OVER! THE FEDERATION OF RUSSIA SEES MICHAEL AND SAMANTHA MORGAN AS POSITIVE PARENTS FOR NIKITA APASTLOV.

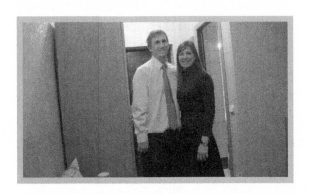

I THOUGHT SO little about the infertility that brought us to this point. It hadn't stopped me from becoming a mother. It had only changed me for the better. I was stronger in so many ways and closer to God, who already had this amazing plan worked out. This was the first time in my life I actually saw God at work; I could see this miracle play out. In a way, infertility was the stepping stone to becoming a mother.

"Are you about ready? Egor will be here in about 15 minutes." Michael's question snapped me back to reality. We were spending the day with Egor, a foreign exchange student from back home, who just happened to live here in Kaliningrad, Russia.

"Yeah, I'm ready!" I called back from the bathroom. How amazing is God to provide such a great kid that we knew from across the world? We just found out before this trip that he lived here and wanted to take us sightseeing. I chuckled to myself as I grabbed the peanut butter Egor had requested from the states.

We spotted him in the lobby right away. I waved and held up the goods we brought for him.

"Aaaa, peanut butter. Thank you!" Egor greeted us. He shook Michael's hand. "My dad is going to drive us around today. It's cold, but are you okay going to the Baltic Sea?"

"Absolutely, we have all day!" I said.

It was so nice of Egor's father to drive us around. He didn't speak English, but I could tell he was so proud of his son. As we drove through the city, Egor pointed out the apartments his family lived in.

"That is one big difference when I lived in America. Everyone had their own house," Egor said. "Most families live in apartment buildings."

"What do your parents do?" Michael asked.

"My father is doctor and my mother a lawyer. I will go to university for law soon," Egor said. I thought about how a doctor and lawyer would live in America. Probably in a gated community with a huge house. Kaliningrad was large, but it wasn't a major city by any means, there was room for houses.

We were soon heading away from town. Not the familiar open fields toward Gusev, but surrounded by thick woods on each side of the road. After about an hour, we pulled into an empty parking lot. It didn't look like much, most parking spots were empty.

"We are here," Egor said.

The wind was brutal, biting my nose as we reached the top of the hill. Below us lay flights of stairs, leading down to the Baltic Sea, zig zagging back and forth. The overcast and fog kept us from seeing far, but it reminded me of the ocean, and I'm sure it's beautiful in the summer. By the time we took pictures and admired the view, we were freezing.

Back at the top was a hot cider stand and a quaint little gift shop. I was always on the lookout for souvenirs, and the shop had plenty of amber jewelry. Because it produced much of the world's supply, amber was abundant here by the Baltic Sea.

"Look, a Christmas ornament, Michael." I picked it up, showing it off. I've collected Christmas ornaments from our travels since our honeymoon to Niagara Falls. Egor was there waiting to help as I checked out with my treasures and thanked the cashier, "Spasibo."

"You said 'thank you.' Where did you learn that?" Egor asked.

"I'm trying to pick up the language," I smiled.

As we traveled on, Egor told us an old Russian tale about why boots were hanging from a bridge we drove past. Egor's dad pulled off the side of the road onto an unmarked dirt path. We followed a short trail that opened up to a retired German WWII tank and underground bunker. Totally open to the public to a point, the cave stretched on past the iron gate. The sight and smell of entering such a historic site was powerful. Artillery and machinery still littered the ground, ready for battle. Outside, we climbed the massive tank to pose for pictures as my hand froze to the metal. Fresh flowers attached to the gun barrel served as a memorial.

We reached the city just before dark, and his dad dropped us all off near our hotel.

"Have you been to the mall?" Egor asked.

"We didn't know there was a mall," Michael said, so we followed Egor across the street to a nondescript building.

"How do you know where everything is? There are no signs," Michael asked.

"There are signs, you just cannot read them," Egor laughed. Down the escalators a group of young boys were horse playing and accidentally kicked Michael.

He looked back, and the boys realized we were Americans.

"Lzveniti ser." The one said looking down in embarrassment.

We looked at Egor asking, "What did they say?"

"He apologized. They are more embarrassed because you are American."

"How can they tell?" I asked.

"You look and carry yourself different," Egor said.

In the very basement of the mall was a grocery store

where we grabbed a few items for our room and some chocolate to take home.

Spending the day with Egor was such a great ending to this trip. From the comfort of our hotel room, I updated the family.

DECEMBER 20,

We spent the rest of the day with Egor, a foreign exchange student at Grove last year. He took us to the Baltic Sea, a German WW2 fort, and around Kaliningrad. We had a great day! We can pick up Rush on January 11th! The only way something can change during the ten wait days is if a family member appeals to the Russian Supreme Court in Moscow! Court only lasted an hour and a half. Tatiana said that court never goes that fast, the judge, orphanage director, and social worker really liked us!

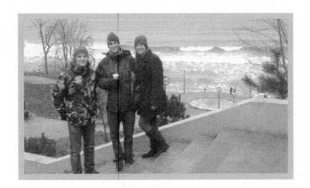

CHAPTER TWENTY-TWO

"Merry Christmas." I rolled over to whisper in Michael's ear.

"Merry Christmas," he smiled.

"Christmas next year will be totally different," I reminded him. He smiled and rolled over, still tired from our trip. We had arrived home from Russia just days earlier. Our Christmas tree shined as a reminder of what was to come this year, and every year after.

"I'll make breakfast," I laughed. I was busy planning new traditions in my mind. Christmas breakfast with all the fixings. The smell of bacon coaxed Michael from bed.

Taking a deep breath he said, "Smells good."

"Thank you."

"Do you think you overdid it on the presents?" Michael asked. Big presents, little presents, and everything in between spilled out from under the tree, while the stockings hung full to bursting.

"Nope," I smiled. I would not apologize for my excited anticipation. I had waited far too many years for a family Christmas with children, and I wasn't about to wait another year. We had spent our life savings and then some on this adoption, so Michael knew none of those gifts were for him. We had already agreed on no gifts for each other and decided to have our Christmas day after Rush came home.

That little voice in my head was still reminding me it wasn't final, reminding me that his biological family could appeal the adoption. I knew it was irrational to think anyone would appeal to the Supreme Court in Moscow, but it was possible. December 30th would be the day I could breathe easy and know that it was final, and know that I had a son. We would leave January 8th, pick up Rush on the 10th, and be home forever on the 14th. The next morning, that would be the first family Christmas in the Morgan house.

Christmas festivities with family were better than ever. Everyone was excited, and I had a hope like never before. A hope filled with peace while I waited. Each day closer to the 30th brought relief, and God was ever soothing.

Thank you, Lord, for your gift of Jesus. You sent Him, your only son, knowing His purpose in life was to die on the cross for my sins. We celebrate the birth of Jesus, and I thank you for the gift of our son. May we teach Rush and raise him to love and know You. Hold Rush tight for me and keep your protective arms around him. Thank you, Jesus.

My favorite room in the house, the nursery, was still

destroyed and needed fixing. I surveyed the green room, and my eyes captured the toddler bed waiting for Krishina. I sat beside the bed and cried, soft tears of mourning rolled down my cheeks. I had yet to grieve their loss, but I had an understanding that they were in a good place.

When I was in college, I remember watching my grandmother suffer through cancer, losing her hair, her health, and her spirit. She was in pain. Her lungs would fill with fluid and have to be drained. When she passed, I was sad, but I knew she was in heaven. She was better off where she was than living in the pain of this world. I sat on the floor mirroring those same emotions. Regardless of what life would or could have been for Yegor and Krishina here with us, they are in a better place with their aunt than in the orphanage. I was sad, but could rejoice in the fact they were out of the orphanage and with family.

Rush would love the colorful circles on the bedding, and I had been working on a crochet blanket of the same colors just for him. One simple tool raised the mattress and added the front piece to create a crib. God had given me a baby. Rush wasn't a newborn, but still a baby. I would teach him how to walk and talk, use a spoon, and play peek-a-boo. I would get to watch my baby grow and be a part of many firsts in his life.

I sat in the rocking chair, handed down to me by my grandma. I would get to rock him to sleep. I loved being rocked as a child, my mom admitting she rocked me till I was six, until my baby brother was born. I would never let

Rush rock himself to sleep again. I would tell him his story and sing him "Jesus Loves Me" as we rocked. God knew the desires of my heart better than I knew them myself.

"Delight yourself in the Lord and
he will give you the desires of your heart."
Psalm 37:4

I FINISHED the crib and moved on to straightening and sorting clothes. With plastic tubs in tow, I packed away the 4T and 5T boy clothes that would have been for Yegor. Rush would be able to use them in a few years, but right now he needed 18 month clothing and diapers. Yes, even diapers. I never thought I would get a child so young. Rush was a special gift, and I was so thankful.

The Minnie Mouse blanket and pink quilts layered the bottom of the tub, while the tights, dresses, and bows went on top. One final fuzzy purple blanket covered it all. Another tub held dolls, toys, and pink picture frames. I felt at peace, knowing God would give me a little girl one day, and as I packed away Krishina's things, memories of the kids played in my mind. Yegor running into my arms, Krishina's little giggle and snort. These are moments that I will always cherish. Even though we were only together for a week and being a family was only a future plan, it was all still real. A real connection, real kids, real dreams. Just like losing a pregnancy, we had plans for Yegor and Krishina.

The pain of losing them would always be a part of our story, and they would always have a piece of my heart. I rested, knowing that their world would not be turned upside down. They wouldn't have to learn a new language or culture, and they would be able to stay with family.

I found healing in putting the pieces of this nursery back together. I finished the room by hanging the orange picture frames holding Rush's first pictures. His name hung above the crib, along with a personalized painting that only lacked his handprint. It read:

"This is the start of your sweet little story,
The part where your page meets mine,
No matter where your tale takes you tomorrow,
Our story will always read love."

New Year's Eve was soon approaching, but today it would be official. Our ten day waiting period ended, and we could finally celebrate our adoption stress-free. I publicly posted to Facebook.

DECEMBER 29,

Midnight in Kaliningrad, Russia! My little man is sleeping and doesn't even know he has a mom and dad today!!! :)

THIS YEAR WOULD DEFINITELY BE a new beginning and a new adventure for our marriage. After eight years of marriage, we would finally have a child to call our own.

Infertility can destroy a marriage and drive a wedge between husband and wife. Were we different somehow? I don't believe so, but I do believe that we knew we were a team. There was no 'me and my problem' or 'him and his problem.' We prayed and tried our best to trust that God had a plan through our infertility. When Michael questioned adoption, I prayed for his understanding. When I questioned God's plan, Michael picked up my pieces and carried us on.

We had no idea what kind of wild ride God would take us on, or the pain that would come with it. If we had known, we never would have been comfortable with it. Even when I lost faith and trust in what God was doing, God never gave up on me. I also had a husband who never threw in the towel. When I couldn't take anything else thrown at me, I knew I could rely on Michael. When he said, "Why not us? We can handle this," I realized our infertility was not a problem to get past, but a choice to make. We had a choice to wallow in our self-pity, or we could pray and take action, be the hands and feet of Jesus.

We could be upset about what we had lost, or we could see it as an opportunity.

"Even in laughter the heart may ache,
and rejoicing may end in grief."
Proverbs 14:13

AFTER FINALIZING the airfare for our final trip, I laughed at how much money was flying out the window. Making a fourth trip completely blew our budget. After visiting several banks and credit unions, who didn't want to loan money for adoption, we settled on taking out three credit cards to pay for the rest of the adoption. I had to laugh, because what else was there to do, except share the irony with our family?

DECEMBER 23,

Final visa applications mailed off, $786. Final plane tickets purchased, $2750. Ready to head back to Russia January 7th and come home for good with our son January 14th, priceless!!!

CHAPTER TWENTY-THREE

January 9,

We made it to Kaliningrad in record time! Flights went smoothly. Can't pick up Rush until Tuesday morning because Monday is still a Russian holiday, vacation for workers.

I hit send and leaned back in the oversized lobby chair, taking it all in. This would be our final trip. I had a suitcase full of little boy clothes and the perfect Gotcha outfit already in the backpack to prove it.

Just over a year ago, we had started this journey, and to think the month we finished our home study, our son was born. God knew Rush would be waiting for us, and we would have never been eligible to adopt him had we not met Yegor and Krishina first. His timing and purpose was perfect. There was purpose in our pain.

This was the day we had been waiting for, Gotcha Day, and I was so ready to see my little boy. Tossing and turning all night, unable to sleep, I would stare at the hotel crib we requested as a sweet reminder of the little bundle we would be picking up today.

With breakfast in our bellies, Tatiana met us in the lobby. "Good morning, Morgans," she said, smiling. "My dad offered to drive you today, so you go with him and I will see you this afternoon."

"Great," I said as we headed to the street.

I liked Tatiana's dad, he was so jolly. He didn't speak English, so there would be no need for small talk. I rested my eyes for the two hour drive, but when I felt the cobblestone streets vibrate the car, I knew we were in Gusev. I got out our camera, wanting to be ready as the lime green orphanage appeared. *This is it,* I thought.

Waiting in the office felt different. It was crowded, and I could feel people coming in to get a look at us.

The white coat of a worker caught my eye and in came our baby boy. I stood with a desire that had never been quenched until this very moment. The worker lovingly placed him in my arms, never to take him back again. She sweetly rubbed his chubby cheek and said her goodbyes with a smile. I was beaming and couldn't stop smiling. There were no tears in Rush's eyes, but his furrowed brow showed his uncertainty. I wanted to comfort him. Lowering back to the couch, I tucked him in my left arm and caressed his little head, kissing him softly.

"Horosho. Shh, horosho. It's okay, baby. Horosho," I

whispered comforting words in Russian. I had been practicing those words for this very day.

"Dress, dress." The worker stood behind him pointing
to her own clothes, showing me to change his clothes
right away. I nodded, but was surprised at the urgency. I
thought they would want him to spend some time with us
before letting him leave. He hadn't seen us in over a
month. "Da, dress," the worker said again.

I had picked out the perfect outfit for today and knew
Inga and the workers would be watching how I dressed
him. Warm was the appropriate attire and I was prepared
with tiny white and navy trim thermal underwear to start.
Laying him gently on the couch, I reached down in the
backpack to retrieve his first outfit.

When he was completely undressed, I handed back his
outfit to a worker. I knew they would need it for the other
children. After the thermal onesie, I slipped on a tiny
yellow, brown, and cream flannel button-up shirt, as well
as fleece lined jeans to match. There was no time for
pictures, but Michael videoed the whole time.

The room was busy with people coming in and out,
stopping to watch us change his clothes, smiling and
talking to each other in Russian. I hadn't known what to
expect, but this wasn't it. Everyone looked so much
happier today than in past visits. I thought, *It must be a
special day when they get to see a happy ending.*

We had gone through so much to get to this point;
soon to be Mom, Dad, and Son. He was adorable and
strangely calm. I added camel soft sole boots and a yellow

puffy vest while looking around for our next instructions. Inga, her secretary, and a few workers were smiling in approval. They were genuinely happy for little Nikita. He would have a very different life outside the orphanage.

"Aaaaa, da! Krasavchik," Tatiana's dad shook his little hand with a huge smile. I wondered how often he got to help his daughter with work. The workers all waved goodbye, and like most women, had sweet dreamy faces as they held their hands close to their heart.

"Are we ready? Should I put his coat on?" I asked Michael.

"Yeah, I guess!"

"Nothing to sign, no more paperwork?" I was skeptical.

"Nyet!" Inga laughed and motioned toward the door. "Da svidannya."

I grabbed the black coat and red and black striped beanie for Rush's head. "Take a picture before you put the camera away," I told Michael. Rush didn't know to look at the camera, he still wasn't sure what was going on, but I held him up so proudly. With that final picture, we were encouraged out the door.

There was no car seat. No concern for safety. The weight of his little body rested on my lap the whole way home. I breathed him in like a perfume. I couldn't be happier, but I was also concerned for him. He had just lost everything that was familiar.

"Doesn't he look confused, Michael?" I asked.

"Well, I guess so. He is probably hot in all that garb you

have him in!" Michael laughed. "You have no idea what you're getting into, little man!"

"Oh, stop. Maybe he is hot." I pulled off the hat and coat and decided I would talk to him the whole way home. It was getting close to lunch time, and I was getting hungry, maybe he was too.

"I prayed for this child, and the Lord has granted me what I asked of him."
1 Samuel 1:27

CHAPTER TWENTY-FOUR

I t was late afternoon by the time we arrived back at the hotel, and breakfast was our last meal.

"I'm starving," Michael said.

"Me too. We need something for Rush too."

"What do you think he eats?" he asked.

That was the moment I realized we had never asked, and no one offered. "Well, he didn't come with an instruction manual, so we'll just have to try some things!" I laughed.

"Let's grab a banana and cheerios from our room before we head to McDonald's," I suggested. "Most one-year-olds can eat those things, it should be safe. I didn't even think to ask about his schedule or food habits."

We quickly retrieved some items from the hotel and headed to our favorite restaurant in Russia. The only place that actually tasted the same as it does in America, good old McDonald's. We both got our usual Big Mac, the only thing we could read on the menu, and found a seat.

Rush was in a state of amazement. He watched people with wide eyes and held on to me with a death grip. I knew he had to be hungry, but he showed no signs, had no tears or meltdowns.

When we sat down, I opened the banana to let him smell it. No reaction. I smashed a piece into a thick chunky paste and spoon fed him. Rush snarled his nose like it was the grossest thing he had ever tasted and spit it back out.

"Well, he doesn't like bananas!" I giggled. "Let's try a french fry." Again I smashed a fry the best I could. With his tongue hanging out, he wouldn't even entertain the fry. "Maybe a Cheerio. They are easy to chew," Michael suggested.

I popped one in his mouth and waited. It didn't come out, but he didn't know how to chew it either. "He's choking Samantha."

I pinched his already red cheeks to look in his mouth and swabbed with my pinky. The little round Cheerio fell in my lap. His face was red and his eyes wide. I felt terrible. I held him close while giving him room to breathe, so thankful for years of lifeguard training.

"I'm so sorry, baby." We were parents for less than four hours and had already let our son choke on a Cheerio. "Eat fast, we need to go to the grocery store for baby food," I said. "We better start a little slower."

FINALLY, the day was winding down. Rush was fed and happy. He had his first bath, all clean and wrapped in a warm hotel towel. I, however, looked like I had taken a bath with my clothes on. In his white and blue thermal pajamas, he scooted around the floor finding things to get into.

"Rush Nikita, nyet, no, nyet," I said as stern as I could to that sweet little face. He just laughed and continued pulling on the lamp and computer cords until I picked him up.

"I don't think either of you know what you're in for," Michael laughed.

We dimmed the lights, and I laid him in his crib. He looked so content and happy. I snapped another picture, unable to control the habit.

Opening the computer, the day raced through my head. Where do I even start?

JANUARY 10 8:26P.M.

He's all ours!!! They handed him to us, we changed his clothes, and out the door we went! It took longer to travel there and back than it did picking him up! Michael and Rush are both sleeping now. Eating was a little tough, tried to give him bananas...didn't like them, tried a smushed up french fry (I know we are terrible, we went to McDonald's) didn't like it, tried a cheerio...almost choked himself trying to get it out of his mouth. We went to the store and bought baby food...I guess he hasn't had any solid food whatsoever! We'll start a little slower.

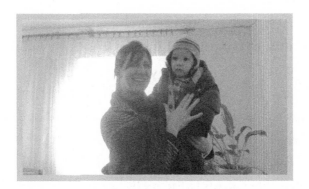

WE WOKE for our final day in Kaliningrad. I wished we could have met our friend Egor one last time, but our time was limited and we would be flying to Moscow that night. When the sun finally rose, we headed out to take pictures with Rush. Victory Square, where the beautiful cathedral resided, would be perfect.

Michael raised Rush in the air with one arm, clearly proud of his son. "I have a picture of my Dad holding me up like this," he said. We captured the square from all sides before returning to the hotel.

"If it wasn't so cold, we could walk to more places," Michael said.

"Someday we will bring him back," I said.

"You can bring him back. This is my last trip across the world," Michael laughed.

TATIANA MET us at the airport along with Allan, Lindsey, and Hannah. "How nice to be able to see my families go," she said.

Tatiana had meant so much to us the past few months, she was a friend. I had a small gift ready for her. It wasn't as much as she deserved, but it was something.

"Thank you so much for everything!" I hugged her, and Tatiana smiled, tickling Rush's little face.

"Idi i delay velikiye dela," she said. "I tell him, 'Go and do great things!'" Tatiana smiled and waved at us all as she turned to leave.

We waited in line with Rush nestled tightly in a sling around my body. I loved his weight next to me, and I planned as much skin to skin as possible. The sling was a little snug, but he sucked his thumb and had no complaints. Before heading on the plane, we snapped a family selfie to remember Rush's first flight and exchanged information with Lindsey and Allan to stay in touch.

Flying with kids was close to first class treatment. They allowed us on the plane first. Resting in our seats, I prepared a bottle for Rush to drink, thinking that may help when we took off. Michael sat in the middle of three seats, his least favorite place. A little old lady stopped at our row and asked something in Russian.

"Angliyskiy," I shrugged with a smile. The woman smiled, understanding that I had said, 'English.' She pointed to a large picture frame she was carrying, then pointed to the ground in front of the seats.

I looked at Michael, "I think she wants to slide that in." He took a deep breath and scooted his feet back.

"Spasibo!" she nodded.

He turned to me saying, "It's a good thing this is only a two hour flight. Did she have to carry that huge thing on?"

"Sorry, do you want to trade spots?" I said.

"I'm fine, I'll just go to sleep."

The flight was quick, and Rush handled it like a champ. He was such a calm baby, and we were in Moscow before Michael even woke up.

CHAPTER TWENTY-FIVE

The doorman took our luggage from the taxi trunk and placed it on a fancy gold cart. We entered the revolving doors into the most beautiful hotel I had ever seen. The marble floors shined all the way to the wrought-iron railing that overlooked a grand piano on the bottom floor. The music from the pianist echoed through the lobby.

"This place is amazing," I said.

"Yeah. Did you know it was this nice? How much was it?" Michael asked.

"I have no idea. The travel agent said it was the closest hotel to the Red Square. Let's just enjoy it. This is our last trip!"

We walked up to the expansive check-in counter, greeted with a smile. "Welcome to Marriott Moscow! Are you the Morgans?"

"Yes!" I smiled back.

"We have a beautiful room overlooking the city and a crib for the baby. Hello, little one!" she said, smiling at Rush. Lifting a finger for us to hold a moment, she lowered behind the desk, returning with a soft brown teddy bear. "For our little guest!"

"Oh, that is so sweet. Thank you!" I said.

"Here are keys, and Alex will help you to your room with your luggage."

I had no idea what a beautiful gift this hotel would be, but I was so grateful. God continued to provide beautiful opportunities and people throughout this journey. Sometimes I was able to recognize the gift, like this hotel or the kindness of a simple teddy bear. And other times, it was harder to see the blessings through the pain, but here we were. We disappeared into the soft king bed before checking out the view of the busy city. The bed felt heavenly; the whole room was beautiful.

The hotel had a wonderful restaurant that we took advantage of. Either motherhood was a piece of cake, or I had the best baby in the world. Rush ate with his hands up, like he was being arrested, and never touched the food or tried to feed himself. Besides his giggles, he didn't cry or complain. He played on the floor or in the crib, and when we laid him down for a nap or bed, there was never a fuss. If he wasn't tired, he laid there anyway. He was wonderful, too wonderful. It was a little concerning. I knew, this couldn't be normal.

JANUARY 11

Rush did so well on the plane! Tomorrow he has a doctor appointment at 6:00a.m. in our hotel room lol! And then the agency goes for us to the embassy to make our appointment on Friday. I think we'll walk to the Kremlin tomorrow afternoon. Our hotel is only a 20min walk. Michael is so wanting to see Lenin's tomb :) Not as much snow here as I thought there would be...just a few inches.

AT 6:00A.M. on the dot, we were opening the door to the doctor. He was kind and attentive, giving Rush a physical.

"You have a healthy little boy here." He was an American doctor working in Russia. We talked about vaccines and other concerns. "Thank you for coming," I said, as he packed up his black medical bag and bid us farewell.

We could tell from our window view the morning was cold. There was dirty snow piled along the streets, but we were determined to get to The Red Square. How many people actually get to experience The Red Square, Lenin's Tomb, and Saint Basil's Cathedral outside of the movies? No, this would be a once in a lifetime adventure.

After breakfast, clothing was layered on like an onion. I grabbed the baby sling we had brought to make the trip easier. It was snug when we used it on the plane, but using it beat carrying him the whole way.

The front desk pointed us in the right direction. "Out front door, turn left. It is straight there, maybe mile, two mile," she smiled. "Must see, most beautiful place in Russia."

Michael asked again, "It's walkable?"

"Oh yes, you can walk there!" she assured us. "Stay this sidewalk, it ends at square." We thanked her and headed toward our next adventure as a family of three.

"I'm going to put him in this sling so he is easier to carry." I threw the sling over my shoulder and around all the layers of my clothes, it was so tight. I could tell this wasn't going to work, so I took off my coat to try again. It was still a little tight, but I lifted Rush up to tuck him in. He wanted nothing of it, kicking and squirming away. This was the closest to a fit he had ever thrown.

"I don't think he wants back in that thing!" Michael said.

"Well, it is kind of small for him. We can just carry him; she didn't act like it was very far." I left the sling on just in case he changed his mind, threw my coat over it, and we set off.

The sidewalk was so busy. I led the way, holding Rush with Michael straight behind, crossing one block after another.

"This is not just one or two miles away! Rush feels like a twenty pound bowling ball!" My feet were dragging, surprised to be the first complaining. People's shoulders brushed one another on the narrow sidewalk. It wasn't as cold as I thought it should be for Moscow in January, but

my toes were starting to get cold. The one place I didn't
have multiple layers.

"I offered to carry him," Michael reminded me.

"I know, but he wants me," I smiled, enjoying being
needed.

"Yeah, and you love it!" he laughed.

"Yes, I do, but here, I can't do it anymore." I handed
him over and Rush never missed a beat. He was wide-eyed
and going with the flow, as long as he wasn't trapped in
that sling!

"We better get there soon. I have flat feet, remember!"
Michael said.

After what felt like an eternity, there was light at the
end of the busy street, and literally, a gigantic red wall
emerged. A massive red castle hovered over the thirty
foot tall arched entryways that were dwarfed by the
building. The intricate white details of each window
popped against the red walls. Delicately anchoring it all
was a beautiful teal Catholic Confessional, adorned with
gold statues and topped with a gold angel holding a
cross.

"It's just like the movies!" Michael looked in awe.

"It's amazing. Go stand over there with Rush, and I'll
take your picture!" I positioned them in front of the teal
room.

We entered the massive red arches that had to be
twenty feet thick. The tunnels opened up into the expansive courtyard. We walked past two characters dressed in
traditional Russian attire, clearly selling photo opportuni-

ties. Each snow-dusted, black granite cobblestone on the ground was hand laid.

The New Year and Christmas season would soon be coming to an end, but everything was still decorated accordingly. A large ice rink was constructed to our left for the festivities, and a white wall surrounded it only chest high, allowing us to see the skaters. Everyone was enjoying themselves. A father was holding the hands of his small child. Teenagers were laughing while leaning against the wall. Laughter filled the square. This was very different from what I expected.

From the center of the square, we could take everything in. We didn't know where to look first, but directly ahead was the famous Saint Basil's Cathedral, the most iconic architecture in all of Russia and a symbol for the country. Legend says the architect who designed it was blinded after its completion so he would never build anything so beautiful again. It stood alone at the head of the square like a beacon.

To the left, past the ice rink, was an official looking building, everything three to four stories tall. Nothing much to look at other than an off white stucco building with a green roof. People were coming and going from inside. With a closer look, storefronts and commercial signage lined the windows. We later learned this was the GUM department store, or what we would consider a mall.

To the right of the cathedral was the Kremlin, fortifying the city from possible attacks from the Moskva

River. Its red walls wrapped the entire eastern side of the square and continued around the corner. In front of the Kremlin walls was Lenin's Tomb. Surrounded by a single chain fence, the small building rose up like a pyramid made of red and black granite, LENIN engraved in large block letters over the doorway. Evergreens guarded the tomb like little soldiers as people gathered around.

The ground was beautiful black cobblestone, shining from the melted snow. We stood in awe of every corner of the square, realizing we hadn't turned around. A beautiful red castle shined in all its glory at the entrance we had just walked through. The same red stucco as the entire surrounding, this was truly a red square. We took in every aspect of it: the architecture, the smells, the people.

I felt a love for these people and their culture. They are just people. God loves these people on the other side of the world as much as He loves me and my people. Governments and wars make us distrust and even hate other countries, but every country is made of people. Normal people. People ice skating. People celebrating the holidays. People sipping hot cocoa with loved ones. People sightseeing. People traveling to work. God loves each one of us.

"This is breathtaking," I said.

I started posing Michael and Rush for pictures to capture it all. First, a selfie and pictures with the cathedral in the distance. I held Rush proudly in front of the iconic cathedral when Michael interrupted with his new favorite thing to say. "You have no idea what you're getting into little man," Michael told Rush, yet again.

"Yes, you have said that before," I could only laugh. I was going to enjoy every minute of motherhood, "And we still have Christmas waiting for you at home!" I spoke to Rush.

"I want to see Lenin's Tomb up close," Michael said.

With the worries of adoption behind us, we were merely tourists now. The square was huge, at least the length of two football fields. Lenin's tomb was closed, but we took plenty of pictures.

Walking along the east side, a winding brick sidewalk led us all the way around the Cathedral, so we followed it looking for a way in. Completely alone on the back side, I eyed the snow piles on each side of the sidewalk.

"I'm going to jump in the snow pile and see how deep it is!" I smirked, hoping no one would see me.

"Okay," Michael said, enjoying having his playful wife back. Glimpses of the woman he married were slowly returning. I took a full jump with both feet into the snow-drift, but nearly fell over from the jolt. I must have looked as disappointed as a kid who just dropped his sucker. Michael laughed. "Not what you expected?"

"Not at all!" I had only sunk a few inches into the snow, the rest must be ice. We continued around the path that overlooked a busy street and similar off-white buildings.

"Look at that building, Michael," pointing to the massive buildings lining the west side of the Square.

There was construction work being done to the exterior, but to look more attractive the entire building was covered in a material painted to look like the side of a building; every detail, windows and all, were painted on. This was the same building we saw from the front but never noticed the construction.

"That's crazy! That drop cloth is massive!" Michael was in shock too. It was so crazy we took pictures in front of it.

We walked around the entire Cathedral before noticing people entering the front doors. Glad to be out of the wind, the dark interior quickly dimmed in comparison to the exterior. The age old archways had some modern additions, starting with the glass doors where we stopped to pay the fee. The small corridors were lined with museum artifacts: century old armor, paintings, and scrolls. With such an expansive building, I thought the inside would be roomier, but it was dark, damp, and depressing really.

"It would be nice if we could read what this stuff was," Michael said.

"Yeah, I have a newfound appreciation for reading and writing," I agreed.

We walked the dark hallways until we came to a beautiful picture window that overlooked the square outside.

"Oh, this is beautiful. It would make a perfect picture." I took out the camera. "Can you set him up in the window sill?" I asked Michael. Rush was very stoic, but he was beginning to keep a little grin upon his face. I think he enjoyed the attention.

Before exiting, the small dark interior opened to an intricately painted foyer. We snapped a family photo on the stone stairs and decided we were all tired and hungry. It was time to head back for a nap.

As we left the iconic square, we were swallowed whole by the people going every which way. We knew how far the walk would be, but the streets were more crowded than before. We couldn't walk as fast or see as far.

"I would pay a million bucks for a stroller right now!" Michael said.

"Give him here, I'll carry him for a while."

The hotel seemed even farther away, and the layers of clothes were far too much insulation at this point. Who knew with all the walking Russia wasn't as cold as I had planned?

"This is taking forever, Michael! I'm so hot and hungry, I can't carry him anymore, and I'm about to pee my pants!"

"Let's find a place to eat then," he agreed.

We continued walking for what felt like miles, surveying signs for something familiar. Out of the corner of my eye, I spotted tiny golden arches across the street. "There!" I pointed. "Let's cross the street at the stoplight."

"Where is it?" Michael looked confused; he hadn't spotted it yet. We were learning that a lot of things here were underground, so in the building we went. "A McDonald's. It must be in this building." Keeping the arches in view, I followed the arrows down a narrow flight of stairs.

I could have done without my heavy wool coat right now. Between my coat, carrying Rush, and the amount of people in this tiny space, I was about to have a heat induced panic attack.

"I have to find a restroom, now! Order me anything," I said, turning to leave.

"Do you want me to keep him?" Michael offered.

"No, he needs a diaper change." My words drifted away as I was swallowed by people.

The cement and rock walls were filled with people crammed in like sardines. I followed the restroom sign down another small flight of stairs. Once in the restroom, that was also just as crowded, I was trying to decide how to accomplish everything. I needed to go so bad, Rush needed a diaper change, and we had layers and layers of clothes to remove. A woman beside me watching my dilemma said, "Ya mogu ego poderjat?" She held up her arms to hold Rush and pointed to the restroom stall for me to use.

"Nyet. Nyet. Spasibo," I smiled and shook my head. There was no way I was going to let anyone else hold my baby, especially while I couldn't see them. Finally, a bathroom stall opened.

Inside the thin walls I whispered, "Lord, please help me." A peace cleared my mind and all the busyness around me disappeared. As I took off my coat and the thick sling that Rush wouldn't get in, I was able to regain my composure. Resting Rush on my knees, I changed his diaper first before taking care of my own business.

Having less clothing cooled my body and mind. I pictured Moscow much colder in January than it was today. After food, we could all conquer the rest of the walk back.

Finally in the comfort of our hotel room, everyone could rest and relax. Michael and Rush fell fast asleep, but I took the time to write to our family and friends first.

JANUARY 12,

This morning was rough...had to wake Rush up for the doctor appointment at 6:00a.m., he just napped on and off, then we drug him around Moscow today...he is beat. But oh, the pictures we got!!!! What a crazy place...I think our favorite so far. Our hotel is a 5 star Marriott Grand...there is a guy playing the piano right now in the lobby! So fancy!!! But everyone here speaks ENGLISH!!!

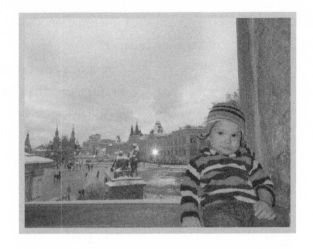

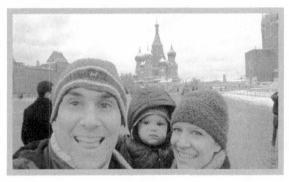

I SHARED a few pictures and took in the amazing adventure this had been before finally taking a well-deserved nap myself.

I was up early again, unable to sleep. The day was planned, with a trip to the United States Embassy. Paperwork had been delivered to us with Rush's Russian passport. I had no idea where things came from or how arrangements got made, but I'm sure Tatiana was still pulling the strings somewhere. With nothing else to do, I checked and updated Facebook once again.

JANUARY 13,

Heading to the US embassy today...we have our appointment to get Rush's visa. His little Russian passport is so cute!

THE U.S. EMBASSY was in a nondescript building marked only with a small American flag. Nothing was special about the outside or inside, except our friends Allan, Lindsey, and Hannah were there.

"How are you guys?" I asked, giving Lindsey a hug.

"We are wonderful! How are you guys?" she replied.

"Great! We went to The Red Square yesterday sightseeing. Our hotel was within walking distance. Well, they told us it was walking distance, but it was pretty far," I laughed.

"Oh, how fun, our hotel isn't close to anything," Lindsey said, "but we went there last time we were here. It's amazing."

We sat together in the white sterile waiting room until our name was called. The government posters and signage reminded us that this part of our journey was coming to an end. We signed a few papers to get Rush's visa and a sealed manila envelope with instructions not to open it, but to deliver it to the customs officer when we landed on U.S. soil.

While waiting for our drivers, I knew this would be our last time with our friends, so we snapped a group photo with the American flag in the background. We traded information and promised to stay in touch.

JANUARY 13,

Rush now has his visa and is ready to head home...he said, he can't wait to meet you all! At the US embassy...see the little American flag on the building. The embassy was the easiest part of the whole thing. We did learn that he will always be a Russian citizen if he wants to be...but if he keeps it, he could be drafted into the Russian army, so we'll be looking into revoking that at age 18.

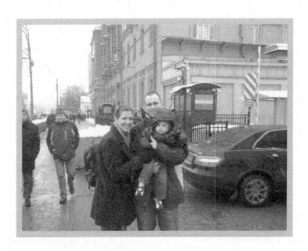

I HAD plans to bring Rush back one day, but would never want him to be put in the army. I remembered our friends Scott and Jenny saying that cruise ships port at Kaliningrad and St. Petersburg. That could be an option that doesn't require a visa to get into the country. Governments make everything so complicated.

Waiting on the oversized sofas, I enjoyed the morning hustle and bustle of the hotel lobby. Opposite of me was a group of men, dressed in business attire having a good time at the bar. It was early morning but they were all drinking, maybe to keep warm before heading out for the day. I got out my camera and secretly recorded their joking and banter. I admire the realness of Russian culture. Nothing is sugar coated. They can come off cold at first, but once they know and trust you, the walls come down. They see small talk and casual smiles as insincere, and I can kind of agree with that. I laughed to myself as I wrote.

JANUARY 13,

We head out at 7:00a.m., the first plane leaves at 11:35a.m. Pray we don't miss the connection in Poland! We should come through customs to officially make Rush a US citizen about 2:00 or 3:00p.m. in Chicago. Will be landing in Springfield at 7:40p.m., hopefully! See you all very soon!

Oh...and pray for Rush's teeth, I think he is teething his 2nd top and has been a bear all day!!!! I don't want that to happen on the planes!

LEAVING Russia for the last time with our baby boy was surreal. Michael was so proud carrying him into the airport. Still new to fatherhood, he sat Rush on the check-in counter for all to see. Unfortunately, Rush was enjoying his freedom more and decided to try to break free. My heart skipped a beat as I watched Rush slip forward over the counter until Michael caught the back of his shirt and pulled him back in. The attendant watched in horror as she took our paperwork. I took Rush from Michael and we walked away, praying no one stopped to take Rush away.

"Did you see the look on her face?" I said.

"Yeah, she was probably wondering why anyone gave us a baby," Michael said.

"US? You mean, gave YOU a baby!" I laughed.

Flying from Moscow to Poland, we were again treated like first-class passengers, being allowed to board first, stewardesses paying attention to our needs. Maybe it was different or maybe it was just my imagination, but Rush was so handsome, people took notice. A sweet older woman with her gray hair pulled back spoke to me in Russian and pointed to Rush. I smiled and shook my head, "Ya ne govoru." I pointed at Rush smiling, "He does."

The woman smiled at him and spoke in a sweet whisper. Rush looked at her mesmerized by her words and smiled as if he knew just what she was saying.

We landed in Poland with a layover before the long flight over the Atlantic. We took every opportunity to give Rush everything he had been missing, and this would be the perfect place to learn how to walk. Michael held the video camera while I held those two little hands. Already so amazingly attached to each other, Rush held tightly to my fingers, as if never to let go.

We walked and talked and looked at everything, making the layover fly by. Before we knew it, we were boarding for the fourteen hour flight home.

CHAPTER TWENTY-SIX

Landing at Chicago O'Hare International Airport was the best feeling in the world. We passed through customs in record time and headed straight to register Rush as a US citizen.

"Hi, we have paperwork for you!" I said, maybe a little too energetic for the officer. He barely looked over his desk and took the papers with an arrogant smirk. I sat Rush up to prepare for a picture.

"Can I take a picture of you stamping that?" I asked.

"NO. You can't take pictures of customs workers," he said.

"Well, how will we remember this day? What can I take a picture of?" I asked, clearly irritated by his comment.

"I don't know. There's a sign there." He pointed with his pen. So we snapped my favorite picture of Rush thus far. His papers were stamped and off we went, running for our last flight home.

Rush should have fallen asleep on the fourteen hour flight from Poland, but that would have been too easy. He was too busy moving the little orange bath toy crab in and out of the aisle and seat legs. Running from the international terminal to the domestic, he finally fell asleep, thrown over my shoulder. We were all exhausted, going on twenty-four hours without sleep, and running through the airport had rocked him to sleep.

We reached the terminal with a few minutes to spare. Rush didn't even wake when we passed him off. Finally boarding our final flight home, a short two hours, Rush was still passed out on Michael's shoulder. I was exhausted and might have drifted off a few times.

Reflecting on the past six years, I could see how miraculous this truly was. Only God could have orchestrated each piece of this complex puzzle. From infertility to adoption, God had a way of changing our dreams to fit His dreams for us. That dream included Rush.

As he slept, I gazed at my baby boy and prayed, *Lord, this is far better than I could have ever imagined. He is perfect in every way and perfect for us. Forgive me for my doubts and anger. Forgive me for my lack of faith. You never gave up on me. You pushed and stretched me to my limit, but you never left me. Thank you, Jesus. Thank you.*

Yes, His plan was way better and beyond what I could have imagined. From such anger and hurt, God never gave up on me. He took a hopeless situation and turned it into an undeniable testimony.

We had set out to adopt two children. When we came

to that decision, two children seemed like a lot, but God had other plans. After living two years without family, Yegor and Krishina were finally with their family in Russia. Although that was so very painful for me, God took those two children out of that orphanage. That loss was so great in the moment that I couldn't see past my own heartache, but our heartache was necessary for God's plan.

Bogdana was the perfect gift for her forever family. A family who had also suffered a great loss. And, well, Rush is right where he belongs.

I laughed at the realization of God's perfect plan. We didn't bring home two kids from the orphanage. God doubled our expectations, and finally I could see the miracle that was in the making; this one, just for me.

"Do not conform to the pattern of this world, but be transformed by the renewing of your mind. Then you will be able to test and approve what God's will is--his good, pleasing and perfect will."
Romans 12:2

RUSH SLEPT the whole flight home. We waited to be the last off the plane and took our time at the restrooms. A stewardess greeted us. "We didn't even know there was a little one on the plane, he was so quiet!"

"Oh, thank you I said. He has had a long trip home," I said.

"We saw such a crowd of people out front, they must be waiting for you! We tried to think of something to commemorate your arrival. Here's a little token to welcome him home." She handed me a pair of flight wings and as she gave me a hug, I began to cry. "Congratulations!" she said. I was overwhelmed by her kindness and the reality that we were finally home. We thought our parents would meet us here, but a crowd of people?

"Thank you so much," I smiled.

Rush looked around from his long nap in a new world. He held on tight as we walked toward the final airport gate. Michael carried all three of our backpacks and just past security, we spotted our families. The green and blue balloons and signs saying WELCOME HOME caught our attention first. We crossed the security line so the welcome home party could meet the Morgans: family of three.

Tears fell as I looked at each waiting face. Each face that had been a part of this journey through prayer and excitement. I stopped short of the group and bent down so Rush could stand. My Dad, as always, had his video camera in hand so as not to be in the middle of the action, but I'm sure he had a plan for after. Mom came first, bending down eye to eye with us. With tears in her eyes and an outstretched hand toward Rush she said, "Hi there."

"Hi, Grandma," I smiled. I could see the yearning in

Mom's face to hold him, but he clung so tight to me she hugged me instead. "I'm so happy for you."

Beside us my brother Curtis grabbed Michael's shoulder, congratulating him as any new dad would. The closer all the aunts, uncles, and cousins gathered, the tighter Rush held on. I stood to make him more comfortable. Michael's parents, Grand Bren and Papa Todd, stood waiting their turn patiently. We went to meet them, "Don't be shy," I smiled.

"I was watching your mother. There is something special about your first grandbaby," Brenda said with tears streaming down her face. Always seeing the importance of every moment, she had waited so my mom could enjoy meeting her first grandbaby. We all laughed and cried until they were about to kick us out of the airport.

"Have you guys eaten in awhile?" Dad asked. I knew he had a plan.

"No, just airplane food," I said, wrinkling my nose.

"I've got the perfect place," he said.

Rush would soon know the depth of love that surrounded him. No longer an orphan, Rush had a ready-made family. Pain brought us all here, but it was God's miraculous plan that brought us together.

———

WE ARRIVED home just before midnight, and all ended up in the same bed. Between Rush's long nap and the time difference, he was not tired at all. We were up most of the night even though we were exhausted, hadn't showered, and had been awake for over forty-eight hours. We finally fell asleep in the wee hours of the morning, and my thankful eyelids closed in unison.

Soft baby giggles and playful hands woke us before noon.

"Merry Christmas, baby," I said to Rush. "Good morning, Daddy," I smiled. "I'm going to shower and make breakfast."

"We'll be fine, Momma," Michael shared my smile. I headed to the bathroom, smiling ear to ear at hearing those words. After the three of us got around and ate breakfast, we all sat in front of our waiting Christmas tree. Sitting on the floor, I helped Rush open gifts, but just like his birthday he loved the boxes and packages most of all.

My heart was full seeing the floor littered with wrapping paper and toys. This was how Christmas should be: children laughing, proud parents watching, thankful for all Jesus had done. The birth of Jesus was a reminder of his perfect life that none of us could have accomplished, and a sacrifice none of us deserved. As I looked at my little boy, I wondered how God could have sacrificed his son for me. Did Mary know she would lose him so violently one day?

Without Jesus's life, death, and resurrection my tarnished life would stay just that, tarnished, but because of his grace and my acceptance of his sacrifice for me I am washed clean.

---

*"That if you confess with your mouth, Jesus is Lord,
and believe in your heart that God raised him from the dead,
you will be saved. For it is with your heart that you
believe and are justified, and it is with your mouth that you
confess and are saved. As Scripture says,
'Anyone who trusts in him will never be put to shame."*
Romans 10: 9-11

AFTER OUR LOSS of Yegor and Krishina, I had been quiet on my public Facebook page. I only shared details about Rush and our journey in person or on our family Facebook page. I feared repeating the same mistake of sharing our wonderful news, only to take it back.

It was like pouring salt in a wound that was being cut at the same time. I couldn't, I wouldn't, be hurt that way again.

But this day, Rush was safe at home forever. There was no chance of losing him, God had delivered this beautiful boy to me. As Rush napped after his busy morning, I publicly announced our good news and my favorite picture.

JANUARY 15

Newest Official American 1/14/2012 4:26p.m. 13 months old exactly

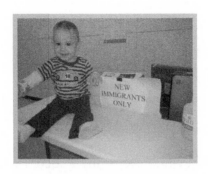

EPILOGUE

Our honeymoon abruptly ended, and the first few weeks were like having a newborn. The time difference wreaked havoc on Rush's sleep pattern. He wanted to sleep all day, and play all night--and why wouldn't he, he was on Russian time. We purposefully kept him awake as much as possible, taking away his morning and evening naps. Within a few weeks, we were all sleeping through the night.

Rush grew very attached to a fuzzy blue blanket he soon couldn't live without. It hurt my heart to see our perfect little boy suck his thumb and rock himself back and forth. He had been alone for so long and had learned to soothe himself. I know his basic needs were met. I know he was cared for, but the love and emotional connection was impossible with so many babies to care for. I spent very little time those first few weeks and months without him in my arms.

The paperwork we received from the baby home was all written in Russian, some even handwritten on small notebook paper. I had friends who knew of a Russian community nearby, and we were able to connect and have those papers translated. This was the instruction manual I needed after picking him up. It contained his schedule and foods he could eat, that was pretty much just oatmeal mush. By now, we had found our own rhythm and plenty of new food to try.

At thirteen months old, he had never had solid food, so baby food was all he would eat for a while. He loved meal time but wouldn't even consider feeding himself. Rush kept his hands up like he was being arrested and leaned in for each spoonful. He was the cleanest eater ever. I could only guess this came from getting his hands slapped or sharing the same bowl and spoon with 5 other babies.

Rush said his first word "hello" within the first month. He was speaking in full sentences and communicating with us by 18 months old. Words came so easily for him, amazingly, after only hearing English for six months. His Russian only came out when he was mad by a rolling R sound when he cried. I knew he was mad, but it was so cute.

His walking and strength grew just as quickly, and he was cautiously exploring his new world. We gave him the nickname "Safety Dan", because he was suspicious and cautious about everything and everyone. Only God knows what our little boy endured his first year of life, but I am so thankful for His loving protection while He miraculously made Rush my own.

"Meanwhile, the moment we get tired in the waiting, God's Spirit is right alongside helping us along. If we don't know how or what to pray, it doesn't matter. He does our praying in and for us, making prayer out of our wordless sighs, our aching groans. He knows us far better than we know ourselves, knows our pregnant condition, and keeps us present before God. That's why we can be so sure that every detail in our lives of love for God is worked into something good."
Romans 8:26-28 Message translation

PICTURES

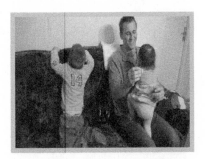

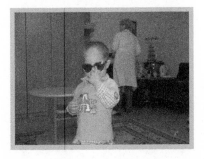

Yegor and Krishina

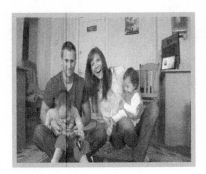

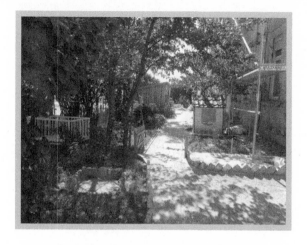

Orphanage Playground

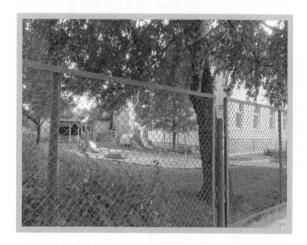

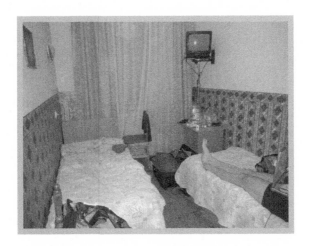

Our tiny, messy hotel room.

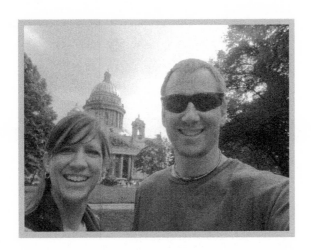

St. Petersburg

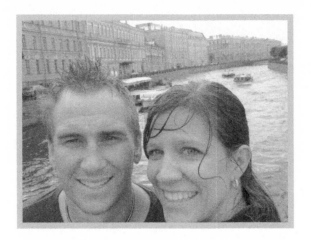

Caught in a rainstorm in St. Petersburg Russia.

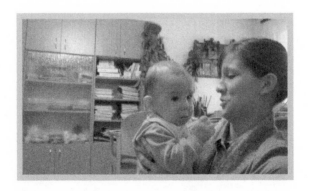

First time meeting Rush

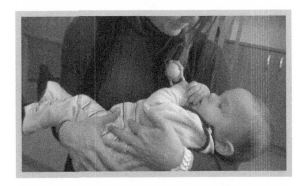

Falling asleep in my arms

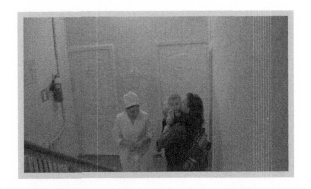

Meeting Rush in the stairwell

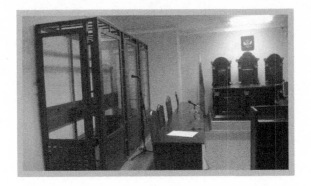

The courtroom

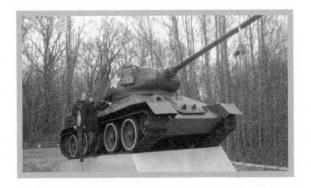

The tank

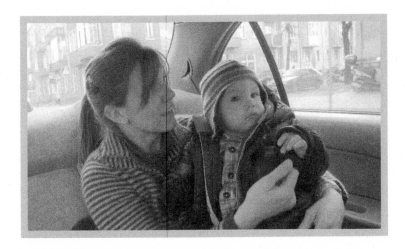

Going home with Mom and Dad.

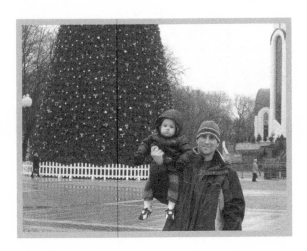

Proud dad holding his boy up in Victory Square Kaliningrad

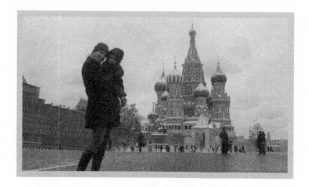

The Red Square

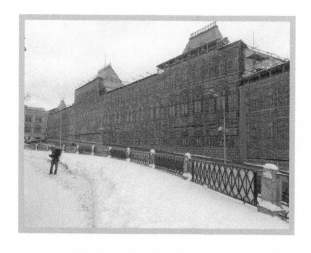

The construction drop cloth at the Red Square

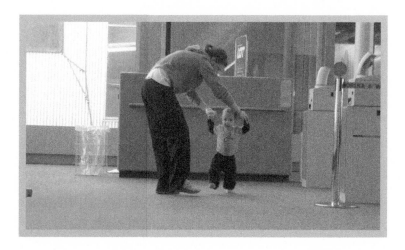

Walking in Poland

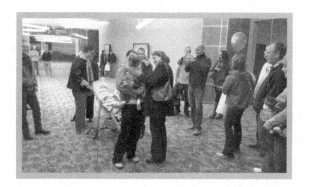

The welcome home party

AUTHOR NOTE

Dear friend,

I share my story so that you too may find comfort in your trials. One day, you will comfort others with your own testimony of what God has done for you. He does not promise a perfect, problem-free life, but He does promise to always be by our side. We may lose faith, but God is always faithful.

A life given to Jesus Christ is a life with hope. If you have not accepted Jesus Christ as your personal Savior, I encourage you to reach out to me or find a Jesus-loving believer to talk to. Because of Jesus Christ's death and resurrection, we have hope that all things, even the painful seasons, have been worked out for our good.

Love and support,
Samantha

"Who comforts us in all our troubles, so that we can comfort those in any trouble with the comfort we ourselves have received from God. For just as the sufferings of Christ flow over into our lives, so also through Christ our comfort overflows."
2 Corinthians 1:4-5

RUSH TO HOPE MINISTRIES

Rush to Hope Ministries was born on Mother's Day 2017 when I shared our testimony for the first time to our church family and launched our website and blog! My goal has always been and still is to connect people by creating a network of beautiful and inspiring stories. I want to connect the people behind those stories with others who are walking a similar journey.

You are welcome to enjoy the blog; laugh and cry with me. You can contact me via email to chat or I can connect you with a mentor who has been where you are. I don't have all the answers, no one does, but having a friend to talk with and have them truly understand is priceless!

If you would like to share your experiences to help others, contact me about writing your inspirational story on Rush to Hope Ministries.

I love spreading hope, and would be honored to speak about our amazing God and overcoming the obstacles of life at your next event. I truly believe the trials in our lives can be a blessing to others.

rushtohopeministries.com
  rushtohopeministries@gmail.com
  Facebook: Rush to Hope with Samantha Morgan
  Instagram: @rushtohope

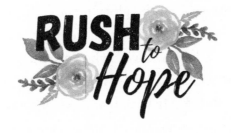

ACKNOWLEDGMENTS

First and foremost, all the glory must go to my heavenly Father for orchestrating such a beautiful story. I am so thankful for Christ's love, who provides above and beyond what is imaginable. He is ever faithful and good.

To my husband, Michael, thank you for pushing me to achieve more, do more, and be more. Thank you for reminiscing with me along this writing journey. You were, and still are, my rock that picks up my pieces, and sometimes, you even tell me to get up and dust myself off. A deal's a deal, I love you.

To my parents, Grandma, and Grandpa; you are the first I call in a crisis, the first I call to babysit, and the first to drop everything to help. Your servants' hearts do not go unnoticed, and I am so thankful to be your daughter. Thank you for teaching me to trust and love Jesus.

To my bonus parents, Grand Bren and Papa Todd, thank you for raising the boy I love and for always believing your "daughter-in-law can do anything". The kids eat way too much sugar at your house, but what beautiful memories you create for all of us.

To my lovely friends woven into the pages of my motherhood story. God brought each of you to me for a different purpose at a different moment. Jamie, Joy, Lora, Tim, Lisette, Lindsey, and Allan, thank you.

To my editors Jessica Barber of BH Writing Services and Kait Craig. There would be a lot less words and a lot more mistakes without you. You both had a major role at different stages of development, and this book wouldn't be what it is without either of you.

Thank you isn't enough for author, neighbor, and now friend, Tara Grace Ericson. God put you in my backyard, literally, to help make this book a reality. Thank you for your never-ending patience of my non-stop questions and concerns. I will forever be grateful. You can find her amazing books at taragraceericson.com.

There are so many people that have had a hand on this story, these pages, and my life. Terina, Ann, Carolyn, Lynn, Sherry, Lori, Donita, Judy, Brandi, Stephanie, Amanda, Yekaterina, my wonderful launch team, and my CCC sisters. I love you all and thank you for being the best cheerleaders.